Passion for Living
a Long Life

Passion for Living a Long Life

◆

How to Prevent and Cope with Ailments

Farzad Tabibzadeh, MD, MSc
Family Physician

iUniverse, Inc.

New York Lincoln Shanghai

Passion for Living a Long Life
How to Prevent and Cope with Ailments

iUniverse books may be ordered through booksellers or by contacting:

iUniverse
2021 Pine Lake Road, Suite 100
Lincoln, NE 68512
www.iuniverse.com
1-800-Authors (1-800-288-4677)

Cover design: Farzad Tabibzadeh, MD, MSc and Siamak Tabibzadeh, MD
No pharmaceutical company, social or cultural organization or any other foundation, has supported this book for publication. The author and the publisher of this work attempted to deliver accurate and current medical information. It is recommended the reader refer to medical textbooks, journals or other sources to obtain advanced information beyond the written medical materials printed in this book.

ISBN-13: 978-0-595-36044-4 (pbk)
ISBN-13: 978-0-595-67321-6 (cloth)
ISBN-13: 978-0-595-80494-8 (ebk)
ISBN-10: 0-595-36044-0 (pbk)
ISBN-10: 0-595-67321-X (cloth)
ISBN-10: 0-595-80494-2 (ebk)

Printed in the United States of America

To all my teachers who supported me mentally and emotionally to become a physician.
To all my patients who shared with me their life experiences.
To my parents, Bahieh and David whose success of their children was their highest priority.
To my brothers, Siamak Tabibzadeh, MD who encouraged me to challenge and overcome the difficulties in life and Farshad Tabibzadeh who was always supportive in my endeavor.
And, to my be-loved wife, Rebeka and my children, Natalie and Limor who supported me during the writing of this book.

Contents

Abbreviations

AA	Alcoholic Anonymous
AMA	Against Medical Advise
BUN	Blood Urea Nitrogen
CAT	Computerized Axial Tomography
CDC	Center for Disease Control and Prevention
CT	Computerized Tomography
CVA	Cerebrovascular Accident (stroke)
DNR	Do Not Resuscitate
DRE	Digital Rectal Exam
DVT	Deep Venous Thrombosis
ECG	Electrocardiogram
EEG	Electroencephalogram
EMS	Emergency Medical Services
ER	Emergency Room
GI	Gastrointestinal, or gastrointestinal specialist (gastroenterologist)
IU	International Unit
IV	Intravenous
IVC	inferior Vena Cava
LDL	Low Density Lipoprotein
NG	Nasogastric tube
PEG	Percutaneous Endoscopic Gastrostomy
PIN	Prostatic Intraepithelial Neoplasia
PSA	Prostate Specific Antigen

SPF   Sun Protective Factor

US   United States

Special Appreciation

This book has been materialized with the significant efforts of my dearest friend, *Mrs. Barbara Butterman*. She is a former teacher and, currently, my assistant. She was a source of compassion and encouragement throughout the years of writing this book. I admire her for her knowledge in helping me with many technical aspects of writing this book. Her dedication is greatly appreciated.

Earning a specific knowledge is more effective

when

your emotions are involved in the learning process.

Introduction

Passion for Living a Long Life contains enjoyable and exciting *true stories* about people who learned from and coped with their illnesses. It depicts their diseases along with their emotional reactions and their attempt to deal with their physical predicaments and how to overcome them. In addition to being a comprehensive outlook on life, this book is an understanding of health and a discussion of medical, cultural, social and medicolegal issues. The stories magnificently present passion, love, loss, despair, and hope, along with mystery, humor, and challenges of day-to-day life. *Passion for Living a Long Life* gives enthusiasm to the insight of a human being in simple terms, making the reader emotionally eager to gain knowledge about medicine and health and learn how to cope with an illness. It is likely that the information in this book will enable people to have a longer, healthier life. This book is a great educational tool to learn how to discuss significant medical problems with a physician. It will also serve health professionals to improve their skills in providing care for the patients.

Unlike mathematical science, which is a straightforward field, medicine engages in complex aspects of emotions of human beings. Classical medical textbooks may describe body organs and the diseases that involve them in simple scientific terms. Yet, besides the symptoms that such ailments cause, people concurrently experience different emotions, including fear when the disease is life threatening.

Passion for Living a Long Life has the following goals:

1. Demonstrating the functions of organs and the harmony that exists in their performance. This book reveals, the thoughts and feelings of the metaphysical nature of human beings and depicts real events in people's lives. The primary intent of the stories told in this book is to greatly enhance the general public's awareness about diverse medical conditions, the psychological turmoil that individuals endure, and how to address both. By the same token, this book intends to guide people toward a healthy life style.

2. Educating the medical community, such as medical students, residents and physicians, about the art of medicine. This book is a didactic tool to teach the young physicians the significance of being perceptive regarding the ones under their care. On the other hand, it is to support many health professionals who already have become deeply involved, both mentally and emotionally, with their patients.

3. Depicting the moral objectives for unifying communities with diversified cultural backgrounds. As a result of ethnical differences, some groups of people may become isolated from each other. This cultural gap may cause disparity or hostility. Unfortunately, in some instances, the end-result may even be bloodshed. Some chapters in this book attempt to pursue humanitarian objectives by closing this gap and making individuals more understandable about ethnical diversities.

The format of the book is designed to deliver the educational and medical information in a pleasant fashion to a variety of people. Most chapters in this book have two sections. The first, and the main section, is the story about one or more patients. The second part contains the commentaries, under the name *Medical* and *Medicolegal Wisdom*, which are based on medical literature.

The tales in this book were inspired by the communications that I had with my patients or with their family members. In each story one or several characters depict some significant medical topics. Throughout the stories, health-related issues from the patient's perspective or as a result of the analysis of my actions as a physician are discussed. Some chronological continuity and medical connections may join one chapter to the next one; however, most of the presented chapters are independent. Therefore, the reader has a choice to focus initially on the parts that are more suitable for the individual's interest. I have exercised the use of a very limited amount of medical terminology in the texts of the stories. Any such terminology has been explained in a footnote or in the list of abbreviations.

The supplemental *Medical* and *Medicolegal Wisdom,* at the end of each chapter, is organized for those who wish to learn more of the medical facts. These sections are presented in simple language. People suffering from a particular illness or taking certain medications may find these sections helpful to enable them to better understand the management of diseases. A general line of explanation was chosen to elucidate many of the medical perspectives. A list of documented references is printed at the end of the book for obtaining further information. The number of each reference correlates with the indicated superscript number in each section.

In summary, the *Passion for Living a Long Life* is a high-quality educational tool for everyone to understand many health-related and medical information through stories. It is also aimed at exposing the human emotions involved in a physician-patient relationship. It would be a valuable source for learning about the wonders in medicine and the art of healing in an effortless and pleasant manner.

1

The Journey

Imagine yourself entering an absolutely dark tunnel. You do not know how you arrived there or how long you may remain in that tunnel. "Where is the end?" you ask yourself. It appears you are not walking, but rather floating and swimming in a fluid. Unclear sounds are frequently heard, but you cannot see where the sound is originating. From time to time, you go under the fluid without any need to take a breath! A small ray of light penetrates the tunnel allowing you to view countless other swimmers around you. They look exactly like you, with a large head, long tail, and no arms or legs. It is true; you are a sperm!

As you continue swimming, a vague opening appears before you. "I must get into that hole," you think. Before you complete your deliberation, the darkness returns. "No!" you say. "I must get back to the track. I must not lose it...Yes, yes, that's it. Here I am. I believe I passed it. Hey, don't push me aside fellow..." you say to the swimmer next to you. "What's all this rush about? Mmm...what's that smell? Probably everyone wants to know about it. It smells so good. But I can't see anything. Let's find out where the smell is coming from?"

A beam of dim green light emerges from the distance. Silently, you keep swimming toward the glow. As you approach, you encounter a very large sphere, radiating the astonishing light that hypnotized you. "I want it," you say. You discover, however, that several of your competitors are already in position to penetrate that shining orb—the ovum. "Hey, get off. It is my turn to go in," you say to the sperm next to you. At the same moment, you push your head into the surface of the ball. "It's piece of cake! This is how you get in...Oh boy. It's harder than I thought. That's why they haven't gotten into the ball yet! I'll lose my chance if I don't enter. Let me try my tail. That's it. I'm gonna make a hole in the surface with my tail and then I'll get in...Come on! How hard can it be? Oh, it's tough. Look at the other fellow. He is jumping up and down on the sphere. No luck for you or for me! OK, you know what? I will swim backward and then try to penetrate the ball with all my force. Here, I'm comi-i-i-ing...No way! It is impossible to conquer this dazzling, glowing sphere. All I can do is kiss you and say good-by."

As you passionately stroke your head on the ball's surface to kiss it gently, suddenly, you feel that you are being pulled inward. "Oh, my gosh! I didn't know the power of love could have such a great outcome. Hey, look! The hue of the sphere's surface is changing to orange. What's happening? I got it. The orb is sealed and no one else can penetrate it. I won! But, that magic smell—It is better than ever. What's this? Another smaller ball? That's where the good smell is coming from. This one will be easier to capture. Let's go in. I love this game. But, but, what's happening. Where is my tail? I'm breaking down. What's that music I hear? La…La…La…Lie…It's a great one. I love it! Where is its source? I'm totally confused. The music again, Fa…Fa…Fee…. Wow, look at the intense coloring of that rainbow bridge. I am fortunate to be here. I am ready to give my all. Let's go to the other side of the bridge and be one. That music is beautiful, La…Li…Li…Fe…Fe…Fe…Fe…LIFE!"

◆   ◆   ◆

Concept of Life

What a great inauguration for two small cells commencing life. However, before hitting the road, let's take with us some philosophical tools about existence.

Your life and mine began when a "smart" sperm among millions of them fertilized one ovum. This was the only opportunity in this world to shape you or me as a human being. However, did you ever ponder why you exist or what life is about? As far as I know, there is no unique response to this question. It took me many years, as a result of caring for people, before I could formulate an answer for myself. In my perspective, life has three basic elements, quantity, quality and purpose.

Quantity—It is the *length of our life on the Earth*. Based on what we carry in our genes, exposure to diseases, or injuries, it can be short or long. Unfortunately, a serious illness or a fatal accident may eventually end one's life. It is imperative to understand that our existence is only a one-time chance throughout the history of mankind. Once you die, you cannot be regenerated. Even through the science of cloning, copying your genes, and duplicating your body, you still cannot be recreated. Therefore, taking care of yourself, as best you can, is usually essential to living long.

Quality—This refers to the *enjoyment in life*. By using our five senses to learn about the environment and by exercising our emotions and functional capabilities we can provide the basis of satisfaction in life. This applies to all ages at every stage of life. Infants may enjoy sucking their mother's breast. Kids take pleasure in running around in the house. Parents are delighted to see their children growing. Members of a family may benefit from sharing, loving, and participating in activities together. And, debilitated, elderly people, whose remaining time will be spent on a wheelchair, may be gratified in having a good meal.

Purpose—Is it enough to improve the quality of our lives solely for contentment, or is there another step that goes beyond self-satisfaction? Answering this question would provide the core to an understanding of our existence. As life goes on and the years pass, we search for an answer, either consciously or unconsciously. Many times, "the purpose" of life formulates and shapes our lives. Interestingly, based on our needs, it is also modified in different ages. The following schematic triangle represents the two elements of quantity and quality in conjunction with purpose.

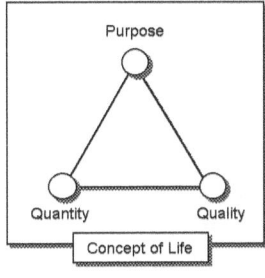

For a human being, the purpose of life can be defined as *obtaining knowledge in order to somehow affect one or more people*. The purpose can be positive when it is beneficial to man and the environment. A father who teaches love to his children, an architect who designs a plan for a building, a president of a company who exercises leadership, are all examples of people with positive purposes. Unfortunately, there are also negative purposes, which are harmful to human beings and their existence.

The "purpose" eventually may influence either the quantity or the quality of life. Depending upon its importance, it can have either a significant or a trivial effect on us. Scientists, who succeeded in producing a vaccine or a remedy for a disease, are unique examples of how they have achieved one of the most honorable purposes of prolonging the quantity of everyone's life. On the other side of the spectrum, Charlie Chaplin was a comedian actor who made people laugh—something that affected the quality of life. In each generation, there are only a few people with truly unsurpassed ambitions. Their impact may be so great that everyone around the globe will benefit from their achievements. These special people, who are found in every scientific or non-scientific field, will have accomplished their ultimate, respectable positive goals and given meaning for their existence.

At this point, I assume you might shake your head and say, "Too much philosophy!" You might be right! But, it is all about fertilization of that ovum by a microscopic sperm and promoting their unlimited aspirations in life—the processes that shaped our existence and the ways we handle day-to-day challenges.

◆   ◆   ◆

My purpose

As a child, I was fortunate to live under the support of both parents. When I was six years old, my mother took me to a pediatrician for a check-up. I remember, from that day on, I wanted to become a doctor. As I grew up, my favorite television show was "Doctor Kildare", starring Richard Chamberlain. The program depicted a gentle, kind medical intern who demonstrated great concern for the well-being of his patients. Then, I said to myself, "I want to be a doctor just like him." Later, "Doctor Marcus Welby Show'" became the center of my interest, because it pictured a family physician who cared for the members of his community. As I became older, I tried to shape my vision and imaginations.

My medical career began in an ancient country, Iran. I attended the only English language university in that country. As a young, enthusiastic student I had a great opportunity to explore a rich Eastern culture in this setting. While I was deeply involved in social issues, the path of my education had to be temporarily interrupted when, in 1979, a revolution occurred in Iran. The new public environment did not allow me to continue my medical career in that country. Therefore, I relocated to Israel, where different civilizations and ethnicities mingled with each other. This transition advanced my understanding about human characteristics. On the road toward achieving higher education, I received my Master's degree in microbiology and completed the medical school. In order to gain a distinctive experience, I joined the Israeli Defense Army as a physician officer, where I learned how to survive under demanding situations.

I pursued my medical career in the field of family practice in the United States. By receiving education in this specialty, I became familiar with a broad spectrum of diseases from pediatric problems to geriatric issues. With such a diverse cultural background and knowledge in medicine, I came to New York, a cosmopolitan city, where I practiced medicine in different settings, such as private office, nursing home, urgent care centers, and hospitals.

I never anticipated that my pathway toward becoming a physician would involve a journey from one country to another. It was a hard and interesting work, full of new discoveries, remarkable people, diversified cultures, and an old but exciting profession, medicine. After many years, the dreams turned into reality. By having a deep understanding of issues regarding various ethnicities, I was able to run my own home-based medical office in a suburban area of New York City. I, Indeed, became a physician serving my neighborhood consist of different ethnicities. Throughout these years, I also inherited a nickname, "*Eddie Tabib*", which will replace my given name in most of the upcoming chapters of this book.

The reality finally took place, but I had repeatedly asked myself about the reason for my existence. As a physician, I try to reach out to as many people as I can through my practice. I follow them very closely and become mentally and emotionally involved with them. However, far beyond my regular duties, I recognized an obligation to offer my knowledge to a larger portion of society in order to achieve a higher purpose.

Medicine is knowledge, which provides the capability of achieving humanitarian goals. This knowledge may have positive effects on the quality and the quantity of people's lives. Learning about health and medicine is an accomplishment of a highly moral purpose. My patients' feedback regarding my care and my past experiences made me believe that there are many people who need to gain more knowledge in medicine in order to have a healthier and a longer life. This is the mission that I chose. Therefore, my path brought me to create a book that raises the value of the existence of each human being and delivers the medical knowledge in simple terminologies to be understandable for everyone

◆   ◆   ◆

Your achievement

I bet as an ovum, when you received that frisky sperm to begin life, you never thought about or planned the years to come. Through the process of fertilization you became a reality, to live and to enjoy life. In addition to the enjoyments, your existence has a purpose—hopefully a beneficial one for the mankind. You are at the verge of accomplishing a new challenge—learning a new perspective about yourself, life, health and medicine. Once you gain the knowledge in the upcoming chapters, you might be able to recognize many health-related problems, learn how to prevent diseases and injuries, or eliminate unfavorable habits. In addition, this information may upgrade the quality of your life by providing you with essential facts beyond mere medicine.

Now, relax and begin taking pleasure in reading about magnificent real life stories of the journeys of many people, including your humble writer. If you are not part of a medical profession, when you finish this book, you may have learned how to prolong your life and that of the others. On the other hand, if you are already in such a field, you may develop skills to positively affect your patients and their families.

2

A Child With Abdominal Pain

You can never predict when you might have to use the information you learned in medical school…

◆　　◆　　◆

Day 1

I had recently established my own private practice when at 7 PM on a cold winter Saturday night I received a call on my pager. After I dialed the number displayed on the beeper's screen, I heard the courteous voice of a man. "Doctor, my name is Michael. My family and I are your new patients. I am deeply sorry for calling you at this hour, but we have a problem with our daughter."

"I hope that I can help," I said. "What is her problem?"

"She developed a rash about 3 days ago, and it doesn't seem to be going away!" he said.

"How old is she?"

"Ten years old."

"Where did you say the rash is located?" I asked.

"On her hands. It really bothers her. I know that it is not convenient for you, but would you please see her tonight?"

"Why is this father calling me on the weekend for a rash on his daughter's hand? Couldn't they wait until tomorrow?" I thought. It was not a convenient time for me to see the girl. However, the idea that she had been scratching herself for the last three days was troubling to me. With this thought in my mind, I agreed to see her. A home-based office made it feasible for me to do so.

Sara was a petite ten-year-old child. She had long black hair. Her "latest fashion" eyeglasses were attention grabbing. She hardly spoke to me when I saw her in my office. Almost all of the conversation was between her father and myself.

She, indeed, had a rash. Her hands were full of signs of irritation due to the itching and scratching. After several questions, I discovered that Sara had received a new soap as a gift from her friends. Once she began using the soap, the rash developed. I gave her a prescription for a cream and told them to call me if the problem continued. I thought that the questions were answered, and the problems had been solved. However, before ending the visit, Michael struck me with a new question. He began, "By the way…!"

As I heard him, the first thing came to my mind was "oops!" Through years of practicing medicine I have learned that this is one of the most crucial statement that a patient may make during an office visit.

"By the way, doctor! My wife told me that Sara has been slightly sick over the past few days. She might have come down with a cold. Would you check her, please"?

I inquired about the cold symptoms or the presence of fever. They were all negative. After I had examined Sara, I still could not come up with any exact answer concerning an upper respiratory infection. I definitely knew Sara did not have a cold. I suggested they schedule an appointment with me for a follow-up visit.

Day 2

Less than 2 weeks later, while I was in my office preparing for the day, I received a telephone call. My assistant called me to the phone.

"Who is this, Barbara?" I asked.

"A mother! She tells me that her child is sick!"

I picked up the phone. An anxious mother began speaking. "Hello, doctor! My name is Eileen. I am Sara's mother. You saw her 2 weeks ago for a rash on her hands. Sara was sent home from school today because of fever. Can you see her today?"

I had never met Eileen, nevertheless, I could identify from the tone of her voice that something was wrong. "OK, no problem! You can come in now. Let's see how I can help you."

Shortly after, Sara and Eileen showed up at my office. It was my first encounter with Sara's mother. Eileen was a tall woman with hazel eyes and black hair. Although she appeared calm at first glance, her anxiety about her daughter was obvious.

After they entered my exam room, I asked about Sara's condition.

"Sara has a belly pain. The nurse in school said that she had a fever, too." Eileen explained.

"Where is the pain, Sara?"

Sara turned her hands upward and shrugged her shoulders saying, "I don't know!"

"Is there anything that troubles you?"

"I don't know. I'm not sure."

I decided to take a shot in the dark. I turned to Eileen and asked, "Does Sara have any nausea, vomiting, or diarrhea?"

"Not really! I didn't notice anything out of ordinary."

"Did she complain of any discomfort when she urinates?"

Eileen shook her head and said "No!"

My professors in medical school taught me that 80% of determining a diagnosis is found by taking a good clinical history. In Sara's case I could not make a firm decision about this dilemma, even after asking a few more questions. So I began to examine Sara. She indeed had a low-grade fever of 99.3° F. Her abdomen was diffusely tender. Since she was very ticklish, like many children, it was difficult to examine her abdomen thoroughly. When I touched her, I was under the impression that she tightened her abdominal muscles. However, when I focused my examination on her back to evaluate her kidneys, Sara suddenly flinched. This finally gave me a clue that she might suffer from a problem in her kidney.

"Doctor, why did she jump?" Eileen asked me quickly.

"Well, she might have an infection in her kidney!" I answered. "But I need to check her urine to get a final diagnosis."

"OK," said Eileen. She looked at Sara and asked, "Can you do it?"

"Aha!" Sara said passively.

After receiving the urine specimen from Sara, I asked my assistant to perform a preliminary test. Surprisingly, the results were not completely consistent with a kidney infection! When someone has a kidney infection, there is usually evidence of the debridment resulting from the battle between the white blood cells and the bacteria. When I received the results of the urine test, I identified a trace of white blood cells! I thought, "Where were the traces of bacteria? If she had a kidney infection, why didn't she have a higher fever? Could it be that I missed something important while trying to make an accurate diagnosis? Above all, why would a ten-year-old kid have a kidney infection?" As I stood in the exam room, looking at the results of Sara's urine test, Eileen's voice cut the silence, "Doctor, is there anything wrong?".

Occupied by a string of thoughts, I suddenly came back to reality. "No! No! I think…Sara may have come down with a kidney infection!" I stuttered. "Starting today, I'm putting her on an antibiotic. But, I want to see her tomorrow!" Then, I gave them the instructions about using the antibiotic. Eileen looked at the prescription and reviewed the instructions with me. Then, she agreed to return with Sara the following day.

After they left, I sat down and looked at the results of the urine tests one more time. "Something is missing here!" I thought. That same evening, troubled by questions of uncertainty concerning my diagnosis, I called my friend, a pediatrician, to discuss Sara's case. After I explained the case to him, he reassured me that an infection in a female child is common and my treatment was appropriate. Although his explanation was very supportive of my decisions, I still was not satisfied. Later that night, I consulted my thick pediatric book. I began reviewing the subject of "pyelonephritis". This is the medical term for the infection of the kidneys. Finally, I believed that I had come up with an answer, as I read, "soap may irritate the genital area of the female child and may cause urinary tract infection."

"Walla! Is this the answer?" I sighed with a deep apprehension.

Day 3

The following day, around noon, Sara and her mother returned to my office. Sara with a shining smile on her face looked happy. With uncoordinated body movements of a child, she was jumping around in my waiting room. She did not appear to be in any distress. Eileen showed her satisfaction by the smile on her face.

"How is our kid?" I asked pleasantly.

"She is just fine! No complaint," Eileen said.

I looked at Sara and asked her, "Well, do you feel better?"

She nodded her head positively, and then putting her hands on her hips, shrugged her shoulders and said, "Yes!"

As I examined Sara, this time she did not react to my stroke to her back to evaluate her kidneys. The fever had disappeared, too! I began thinking, "What a great recovery! Could it be any better than this? Fever is gone. No sign of infection. She is cured! And, her mom is satisfied. They feel that I did a good job. What a great success! All of that, after just one day of treatment with an antibiotic." Suddenly, the last fragment of my thoughts struck me! "…Only *one* day treatment with antibiotic!" My thoughts screeched to a halt! It was too good to be true! Like reviewing videotape, my idea from yesterday rushed back into my mind, "Why in the world would a ten-year-old kid get pyelonephritis?"

"Well, do you know why she got this infection?" Eileen asked.

"Soap! Washing the female genitalia with a soap may cause a urinary tract infection," I explained. Yet, while I was not totally convinced, I tried to sway Eileen, and myself, about what had happened to Sara.

"Soap? Really?" Eileen said with hesitation.

Deep down inside, I had a feeling that something else was wrong with Sara. There was something more, beyond a simple infection of the kidney. Finally, I broke my silence. "Listen," I told Eileen. "I know that she feels better, but I want to do more tests on Sara."

"Why, doctor? She seems fine. Do you think that something is wrong"? Eileen's voice was trembling. Suddenly, I felt that the level of her apprehension was more than I might have expected. Was it my imagination or was it true? For a fraction of a second it appeared that she was desperate to do something for Sara.

"I want Sara to have an ultrasound of her kidneys," I said. "That is a simple procedure. I think Sara can tolerate it."

"OK. If you think so," Eileen said, "I'll call for an appointment as soon as possible,"

"That will be good," I said. "So, I will be in touch with you when I get the report of the ultrasound."

As soon as Eileen returned home she scheduled an appointment for the ultrasound. Michael, Sara's dad, arrived home later. He asked about Sara's visit with the doctor. "How did it go, Eileen?"

"The doctor said that Sara might have an infection of her kidney," Eileen answered.

"What do we have to do for this?"

"He's sending her for an ultrasound."

"An ultrasound!" Michael said. "Is there anything seriously wrong with her? Didn't the former pediatrician say she had allergies? Just like the rash she had on her hands!"

"Allergies! You're right. But, I feel I have to follow this doctor's recommendations," Eileen said.

I don't understand how this doctor wants to connect allergy and a slight fever with an ultrasound? All right. Did you already make an appointment for Sara to have the ultrasound?"

"Of course."

"When is it for?"

"They had an opening for tomorrow. So I made the appointment."

"That sounds good. The sooner the better!"

<u>Day 4</u>

Sara and her mother arrived at the radiology department at 9:00 AM. When Sara was called in, she was asked to lie down on a stretcher for the exam. After simple preparation, the sonographer began scanning on Sara. Eileen held Sara's hand. Sara was staring at the monitor. Numerous white and black spots were displayed on the screen. The sonographer took several pictures. When she finished, she developed the pictures and prepared to leave the room.

"Is everything OK?" Eileen asked.

"There is something! I can't tell you anything more, but I'm sure our doctor will speak to you," the sonographer answered.

Still holding the pictures, the sonographer left the room. She walked down a long hall until she reached Dr. Saffron's office. The door was wide open. She walked straight to Dr. Saffron. He was sitting in front of an illuminated board with a few x-ray films on it, dictating a report. She waited patiently until shortly thereafter the doctor finished his dictation.

"OK. What did you get for me?" he asked as he returned the x-ray films to their large folder.

"Dr Saffron, this is an ultrasound of the kidneys of a ten-year-old child. Do you see what I see?" the sonographer asked.

Dr. Saffron picked up the films and hung them on the illuminated board. As he studied the films, he said, "Oh boy! Who is gonna miss such a finding? Of course, I can see it! Where is the child?"

"She is still here with her mom. Do you want to speak to them?"

"Yes. Let's go to see them," he said as he rose from his chair and walked toward the door.

Dr. Saffron and the sonographer headed toward the ultrasound room. Upon entering, they found Sara sitting on the stretcher. Dr. Saffron introduced himself, "Hi, I'm Dr. Saffron, one of the radiologists."

"Hello. I am Eileen," she said as she extended her arm to shake hands.

"Listen, Eileen! There is something in one of the kidneys," Dr. Saffron said.

"What is something?"

"It looks like a mass!" he responded

"A mass! What do you mean by that? Is this bad?" Eileen questioned.

"Well, we have to see. Your daughter might need to have more tests done. I need to speak to your doctor to see what else we can do."

"Do you need his number?"

"No! We have his number on file." Dr. Saffron explained.

"Will you let us know what to do?" a frightened Eileen asked.

"Yes, of course! I'm going to give him a call now." Dr. Saffron said as he gently touched Eileen's arm with his hand.

Dr. Saffron and the sonographer left the room. Then, as he turned to her, he asked, "Who is the attending?"

"Dr. Tabib," the sonographer answered.

"Get him on the phone for me, please."

It was a busy day for me. I was doing my round in the hospital. Around 10 o'clock in the morning, when I was in the middle of writing a note about a patient, I received a page. An unfamiliar number appeared on the pager screen. I stopped writing and picked up the phone to dial the number. After several rings, a young woman on the other end of the line answered, "Radiology!"

"Hi, this is Dr. Tabib. Did someone page me at this number?"

"Oh, yes! Dr. Saffron is looking for you. Hold on, please."

A moment passed. Then I heard, "Dr. Tabib, Hi. This is doctor Saffron, one of the radiologists."

"Hello, Dr. Saffron."

"We finished the ultrasound on one of your patients. She is a ten-year old child who came in for a renal ultrasound." His rapid but concerned voice stunned me.

"Are you talking about a child named Sara?" I asked.

"That's right."

"So quickly she had the ultrasound? I gave them the referral just yesterday!"

"Well, they acted fast. Anyway, she has a problem!" Dr. Saffron stated.

"What is the problem?" I questioned.

"She has a mass in her kidney." As he said that, my hands became numb. I could not think clearly at that moment. I was as if a thick fog enveloped my lucid mind.

"A mass…Oh, my gosh! You mean she has a tumor in her kidney! That's not good!" I said.

"No! No good at all!"

"Does the family know about it?" I asked.

"Yes. I informed the mother."

"So, she should be worked-up!"

"Yes. I'd like to have your permission to do a CT of her abdomen and her chest," he said.

"That sounds OK to me. Please, go ahead," I responded.

"Very well!"

"I appreciate you're calling me. Please keep me informed about the report," I said.

"No problem. We'll be in touch," he said.

I hung up the phone and began silently praying for Sara. I prayed that the tumor would have a favorable course. For the next two hours, my mind was unsettled because of Sara's condition. As I was struggling to finish my hospital round at a normal pace, a few blocks away, Sara was undergoing a CAT scan. At 12:00 noon, sharp, I received another page. This time, I recognized the number. It was the radiology office. I immediately called the number and spoke to Dr. Saffron.

"Dr. Tabib!"

"Yes! I'm here. Did she have the CAT scan?"

"Yes, she did. It is not good!" The devastation and disappointment in Dr. Saffron's voice echoed over the phone. "This girl has metastases to her lungs!"

I paused in our conversation, and then I asked, "In the lungs! Did you notify the family this time, too?"

"No! They don't know about this part."

"Well, I believe I have to talk to them," I said.

The ominous concept of "metastases", as an already advanced disease, was clear to me, but not to Sara's parents. Therefore, moments after I ended my conversation with the radiologist, I called my secretary to arrange a visit with both of Sara's parents later that same day. Upon returning to my office, I realized I had mixed emotions about this task, which laid ahead of me. I had feelings of fulfillment about successfully defining a difficult diagnosis, but I was burdened with despair over Sara's condition. I recalled the first time Sara came to my office. It was only for a simple allergic rash. I recalled also her father's "by the way" question…about "slight sickness" that Sara had on that day. With such an advanced disease, Sara had been sick for a long time! Why wasn't she diagnosed earlier? Why hadn't I made the diagnosis on that cold Saturday night during her first visit? What was the obstacle? I realized complaining about the rash was a factor that masked another major problem. Her superficial quick recovery after taking the antibiotic was another ambiguous component.

At five minutes to 2:00 PM, Sara, along with her parents, entered my office. Sara looked happy. She did not have any clue about what was happening to her.

After a briefing with her parents, I asked Sara to come to the exam room. I invited her to recline on the examining table for a final evaluation before breaking the news to her parents. As I tried to check her abdomen, she was still ticklish and displayed a firm abdomen. Finally, I calmed her down. Then, I was able to perform a revised abdominal exam. Positioned *very deep* in her abdomen, there was some "firmness". It was a finding that could easily be missed by any physician, due to its location and the *involuntary reflexes* of Sara's abdominal muscles.

I was very anxious about the meeting. Although I had ample experience in notifying patients with unfavorable test results, this situation seemed more difficult than the others. Telling parents that their ten-year-old daughter was suffering from a serious illness, which may even lead to death, was not easy at all! I tried to put my emotions aside to focus on the conversation I planned to have with them. I expected the meeting to be painful. To encounter such an occasion is difficult for any physician, regardless of earlier preparations.

I asked Eileen and Michael to come to my consulting room. They sat next to each other. Sara was directed to sit in the waiting room. As I took my seat, my heart was pounding. I looked at them and then asked. "How much do you know about the results of the tests?"

"The radiologist said that she had a mass in her kidney," said Eileen.

"Well, that's correct. But, it is more than that!" I explained. "Unfortunately, the news is not good. It is a tumor which has spread to other parts of her body!"

"What do you mean by spread?" Eileen appeared confused. Michael rubbed his forehead, and tried to focus on the conversation.

"I mean she probably has cancer that has invaded other parts of her body," I calmly explained.

"Cancer!" Eileen's eyes became tearful. Michael compassionately placed his hand on her arm for support. Then, contrary to my understanding, I discovered that their knowledge about Sara's condition was less than I thought. It was at this moment that Eileen connected the word "mass" with "cancer"!

With a gentle voice Michael said, "OK! OK! Take it easy! Let's see what is going on here." He desperately tried to keep his wife calm by gripping her hand. "How far has it spread?" he continued.

"Unfortunately," I said, "it has traveled to the lungs."

"Any where else?" Michael asked.

"No! Not as far as I know," I said.

"How long do you think she has been suffering from this?" asked Michael.

"My guess, for a long period of time!"

"Weeks? Months?" asked Michael.

"Probably months."

"But," Eileen said, "We were told that she was suffering from allergies!"

This information stunned me. I remained motionless for a second. Then I asked, "Who said that?"

"The previous pediatrician! Sara has been having these episodes of being feverish for a while!" said Eileen.

"Feverish? How long has this been going on?" I asked.

"For about 3 to 4 months," Michael answered.

"Three to four months!"

"He kept telling us that she had allergies," Eileen said.

"Allergies!" I said. It was then I put the pieces of the puzzle together. Changing to a new primary physician, a desperate visit to a doctor's office on a Saturday night, the history of a "slight sickness", rushing for an ultrasound without any delay, was all the result of a their long-term concern about Sara's condition.

"Well,…this is in the past. What are we going to do now?" asked Michael.

"Sara probably needs surgery. This means a resection of her kidney. She might also need some chemotherapy. At this point she needs a urologist and an oncologist."

"When do we have to see them? Tomorrow?" asked Eileen.

"No! Today," I said. "Let me call the oncologist now."

Eileen and Michael were at the most desperate point of their lives. I could read the sadness and devastation in their eyes. It seemed, without warning, a fog of uncertainty had surrounded them, making it difficult to think. They needed guidance and direction. For consolation, I asked them to remain in my consultation room. I dialed the telephone number of the pediatric oncologist with whom I was acquainted. Michael began pacing on the floor. Eileen resembled a severely emotionally wounded person as she cried softly. My conversation with the oncologist was brief. He was very understanding about the situation and agreed to see them that same afternoon.

"Listen, let's pray for the best," I said. "Go and see the oncologist now. He will give you more information about what we need to do. Let's take it one step at a time."

"One step at a time!" repeated Michael anxiously, "God help us!"

They headed off to the oncologist's office. I was left with haunting thoughts. Sara had been sick for the last three to four months, or probably longer! I had the impression that Sara's parents left the previous pediatrician because they sensed Sara was suffering from something more than "allergy". What would have been the outcome if I had never checked her kidneys? I remembered when she flinched during examination. What if I had not been suspicious about the results of her urine test? What if I had not trusted my gut feeling about the ambiguous diagnosis, which eventually led me to request an abdominal ultrasound? Sara went for a test, the results of which had significant effects on her life and the lives of the people around her. She was a 10 year old with many dreams. This test altered the course of her destiny and also that of her parents. Sara could have possibly gone on without a definitive diagnosis and without any intervention if I had relied on the one-day treatment with antibiotic. Outwardly, she had an overall healthy appearance, without any significant symptoms of malignancy.

After the oncologist examined Sara, he decided to hospitalize her the same day. The plan was an immediate resection of her kidney by a pediatric urologist!

Day 5

I went to see Sara on the pediatric floor of the hospital the next day. Sara was hiding under a red hospital blanket. The colorful wallpaper with Disney characters was eye-catching. Several people were in the room. I recognized only Eileen and Michael. The rest of the people, I later learned, were close family members. In two hours, Sara was scheduled to have the contemplated procedure to remove her diseased kidney.

The entire family looked deeply depressed. Eileen was standing just next to Sara's bed, trying to take care of her quietly. She glanced at me, but did not seem to have any interest in making conversation. I approached Michael. He was still in shock about what was happening to his child, but he appeared more open to exchange ideas. We talked briefly about the different types of kidney tumors and the various options of treatment. He already knew about Wilms tumor and Neuroblastoma. However, our conversation was far from complete because of his heavy emotional state. He asked me question after question, trying to imagine what the future held for Sara. It was very difficult for me to answer regarding the uncertainty of Sara's destiny. In the end, I found myself becoming extremely emotional. I gently held Michael's right hand and said, "Good luck!" He looked directly into my eyes and said, "We trust in god!" Eileen was sitting almost motionless in her chair, next to Sara's bed. I could not find any strength in myself to approach her to say a farewell. I did not want to disrupt her silent moment. I looked at Sara once again, and then, to regain my composure and objectivity, I left the room quietly.

In the next few days

After Sara's surgery, her family and I were anxious to learn the final diagnosis. We were praying for good news. I was hoping the diagnosis would be a Wilms tumor because of its more favorable prognosis. Would it be Wilms tumor?

The day after the surgery, when I went to the hospital to see Sara, Eileen and Michael appeared somewhat relieved. This time they had smiles on their faces. Michael said, "They told us that it was probably a kind of Wilms, but still don't know about the aggressiveness of the tumor". Michael was referring to the preliminary pathology report. The final report would be available in two or three days. We just had to wait.

Two days later I received the final report from pathology. It read, "Well differentiated Wilms tumor!" This was good news. Finally, the beast, living as a metastatic cancer in Sara's body, was identified! There was a ray of hope that it could be beaten with chemotherapy. This meant a long battle with cancer. Anybody who has had treatment with chemotherapy knows how difficult it can be—especially for a child.

Although Sara had a chance for recovery, death was still circling above her head. The family agreed to proceed with chemotherapy. Sara had to undergo another procedure to install a small intravenous port (IV-port) under her skin. For a long-term device such as this, there would be a risk of infection as long as it remained in her body. However, this was a "manageable" risk that Sara had to take.

The next few months

It was necessary for Sara to interrupt her education to receive chemotherapy on a weekly basis. Eileen obtained a home tutor for Sara to assist with her studies and prevent any lapse in her schooling. These were drastic changes in Sara's life. One surprising and joyous event occurred in Sara's family soon after her diagnosis. Eileen became pregnant! In Sara's private world, she wished to stay alive long enough to one-day holding the baby!

Since Sara was mostly under the care of the pediatric oncologist, I did not actively follow her after my initial assessments and referrals. However, I received all of the progress reports during her treatment. It was emotionally difficult for Sara, especially right at the stage of becoming a teenager, to deal with many of the consequences of the chemotherapy. They ranged from her hair falling out to becoming nauseous at times, and having a blood test after each of the sessions of the treatment. All were arduous for her and her mother.

Seven months into therapy, Sara was required to have a CAT scan of the chest to track the progress of the metastasis. The report was promising. At last, there was absolutely no trace of metastases in the chest! This was the best news for Sara after quite some time! The entire family celebrated that night. However, the nightmare of chemotherapy would have to continue for another few months.

Two months later, Michael took Sara and her younger brother, Robert, to the hospital. This time it was not for Sara. As a matter of fact, they were going to see Eileen. They wanted to see the new baby, Jonathan! Two days later, when Eileen returned home, she received a surprise! Her room was filled with flowers, a reception from Michael that she could never have imagined. Sara also got her wish. She held the baby!

One and a half years later

Spring brings many new beginnings. I was at home one day in early April. My two little daughters, who were playing in the yard, had been amusing me. Suddenly, the telephone rang. My wife picked up the phone and, after a brief conversation, she handed it to me.

"Hello!" I said.

"Dr. Tabib. Hi. This is Eileen, Sara's mother."

"Eileen! What a surprise! How is everything?"

"Everything is good."

"How can I help you?" I asked.

"Is it possible for you to see Sara tomorrow?"

"Sara! Is there anything wrong with her?"

"No! No! We just need a medical clearance from you to have the IV-port removed," Eileen explained.

"Wow! This is the best news that I have heard today! This means that she is finished with the therapy. Is that right?"

"Yes! That is right!"

"It will be my pleasure to see her in the morning," I said.

After the conversation, I marked my office calendar to see Sara early the next morning. It had been a while since I had last seen her. The next day, she came in with her mother. Sara still looked slim, but taller. She appeared more mature, compared to the previous year. I could detect a hairpiece on her head. I was also impressed by her happiness. Although Eileen tried to show some satisfaction, she looked exhausted. I imagined her condition was probably due to the many months of dealing with Sara's therapy.

For me, it was quite a moment of exhilaration to see Sara in good health. Finally, she was free of disease. During her physical exam, I noticed the long scar on her abdomen, which extended to her back. This surgical scar was the result of the removal of her kidney. At the end of the session, I signed a form of "medical clearance" which I probably could have renamed *"certificate of health"*!

After they left, I sat down to ponder what I had witnessed over the previous year. How much must parents do for their children? It is a never-ending battle for their happiness and well-being. At times, it even seems that we live for their well-being. The love that parents have for their children is an unlimited passionate love of one human being for the other.

Four months later

At the end of my hectic day, I was not eager to wade through the pile of mail that had accumulated on my desk. I studied the pile, raised my eyebrows, and thought, "That's it! I'll leave it for tomorrow." Just before I walked away, I glimpsed an unusual purple-edged envelope sticking out of the pile. I pulled it out. Upon opening it, I found a very beautiful card in colors of white and purple inside. It was from Sara's family, inviting me to her Bath Mitzvah! Tears filled my eyes. I wanted to shout with joy, but my voice was trapped in my throat. Suddenly, all of my fatigue of the day was replaced with happiness and energy because Sara had reached to an important milestone of her life.

Two months later, exactly two years and four days since I had diagnosed Sara with Wilms tumor, my wife and I walked into an elegant party given for Sara's Bath Mitzvah. Michael and Eileen greeted us with open arms. At the opening of the reception, Sara was busy with her friends. Many people in elegant evening garments were in attendance. The colorful flower arrangements on the tables made the party very attractive.

When the time came to light the candles, I could see the glory of life around Sara. She was like a shining star on the stage. Although shy, she was filled with confidence. With a radiant smile, she called the names of her family members to come to light the candles. Finally, she invited her parents and her two brothers to light the last candle. Everyone stood up and began to applaud. As I stood with the crowd, I felt a teardrop of joy running down my cheek. I had great pleasure sharing this moment with Sara and her family. It was her destiny to have such a beautiful night. The event was not only a Bath Mitzvah party, but also a celebration of life.

Life is like a boat floating on the sea. It journeys from one port to another. We are the passengers on this boat. At times, the sky is sunny to allow us to enjoy the weather. On other occasions, the sky is rainy and the storm tosses the boat. For Sara, the storm was over. Her boat moored anchor in a safe port.

MEDICAL WISDOM

Fever in any age group is a nonspecific sign of a disease. If the fever subsides over a short period of time, it is most likely due to a viral infection. If the fever lasts beyond a couple of days, it may require a medical work-up. A combination of fever and other signs may narrow the diagnosis.

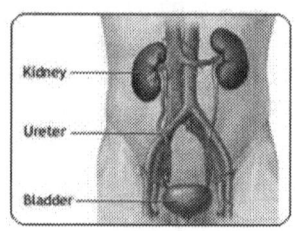

Urinary System

Abdominal pain is either new or recent (acute) or chronic and recurrent in its nature. Location, quality, onset, and the duration of the pain may help the physician diagnose the condition. For example, an acute pain, which originates in the right lower side of the abdomen, and is associated with fever, may be caused by appendicitis. On the other hand, a recurrent pain around the umbilicus may signify a functional problem in a child. This kind of pain may appear in a 5 year old perhaps as a sign of family stress or school phobia. An acute pain originating in the back and radiating to the lower part of the abdomen, with or without fever, may represent a problem in the urinary system, e.g. in the kidneys or bladder.

Malignant tumors in the kidneys are rare in children. The most common of those cancers are neuroblastoma and Wilms tumor. Neuroblastoma is more common in infancy, mostly around 1 to 3 years of age. Most of the cases of neuroblastoma are presented as a hard abdominal mass. Although this disease depends on its progression, unfortunately its prognosis is poor.

Wilms tumor is a rare malignancy in children, with an annual incidence of 7.8 new cases per million children. The mean age of diagnosis is 2–5 years. Wilms tumor rarely occurs in teenagers or adults. In young children and toddlers, parents may discover it incidentally while bathing or dressing the child, or a physician may detect it during a routine well-child examination. Up to one third of the cases of Wilms tumor may be associated with abdominal pain, fever, weakness, presence of blood in the urine, or elevated blood pressure. This tumor, just like many other malignant diseases, can be differentiated at its cellular level. This means that some Wilms tumors are more aggressive than others. It also can spread to different parts of body, such as the lung, liver, bone, or brain. Surgical resection of the tumor, combined with radiation therapy and chemotherapy, are important strategies to cure this disease. The prognosis of Wilms tumor, based on the cellular differentiation and advancement of the tumor, is generally favorable.

For me, Sara's case stirred up memories from my days in medical school. Back in Israel, many years ago, I was going through my rotation in the pediatric unit. A young, energetic, female attending physician gathered our small group of medical students together to teach us about kidney tumors in children. After a very brief introduction, she mentioned the names of "Neuroblastoma and Wilms tumor". In her rapid paced presentation, she explained that both these tumors were extremely rare. Neuroblastoma is found in infancy and Wilms tumor occurs in early childhood, usually between the ages of 3 to 5 years. At this point in the lecture, I remember I thought to myself, "Well, I'll never be a pediatrician. Why do I have to know about these rare diseases? I'll never encounter any one of them in my life!"

It was true I never became a pediatrician, but I became a family practitioner who cares for children as well. In this capacity, I came across a child with this very rare disease. I could have never imagined the information from that lecture would materialize into a human being, who, one day, would sit before me as "Sara", with abdominal pain and a slight fever! Furthermore, this case was extremely rare because Sara was ten years old. She was beyond the age of developing a "Wilms tumor" in her kidney, but she did. As Sara's pediatric oncologist said, "Sara was the oldest Wilms tumor patient he had ever seen during his years of practice". Sara, the person, simply disobeyed the rules of a medical textbook!

Despite the gravity of the situation, and given all the ambiguity that surrounded Sara's case, it was a good judgment for me to follow my clinical impression and order a simple ultrasound to establish her diagnosis. Finally, after many years, what I assimilated from that medical school lesson was "listen and learn!" You would never know, in advance, when you will use what you hear.

3

Healing of a Distressful Incident

The present emerges from a legacy of past experiences and events. So a physician bases the practice of medicine on an accumulation of many integrated emotional memories. In my case, the gratitude that I feel in making the diagnosis of a disease is not without an emotional burden that took a toll on me a long time ago. This is related to the conversation and its unpredictable events following what happened in Tel-Aviv, Israel. The impact was intense enough that it affected the way I practice medicine today.

"…I have an appointment at 12:00 o'clock with Mr. Ariel Sharon, the Minister of Defense," the robust, tall man explained.

"I understand how busy you are," I said. "However, she needs to be transferred to the hospital."

"OK, if you want to transfer her, you have to take her to Ichilov Hospital."

"Sir, I can't transport her to Ichilov. I have to take her to the nearest designated hospital."

"You know what?" he said. "It doesn't matter. I'll take care of it. I'll take her to Ichilov Hospital if I have to do so."

"Sir, are you sure about what you want to do?"

"Yes. I'll take the responsibility," he answered firmly.

◆　　　◆　　　◆

The day I took my last exam in medical school, I felt I had survived the collapse of a ten-story building. This ended ten very intricate years in different schools in two different countries. I was not aware that graduation from medical school was the easy part. I could not predict that the future would be even tougher.

As a physician, I was involved in making decisions about people's lives. It was not only about "how," but, also, about "when" and even "where" to treat them.

The process of treating a patient can be a composite of medicine and law. Problems may arise when the medicolegal system is not followed correctly. However, a physician may become involved with something more influential than the system—guilt! Feeling guilty, especially for a long period, may make a person vulnerable. In some instances, the guilt may force a physician to become a more ethical person when it comes to the care of his or her patients.

The following story is about when I was a young, inexperienced physician back in Israel. It concerns the first time I took care of another human being without direct supervision. It is a story of how insufficient knowledge and skills, along with an unfamiliar environment, led me to experience many years of anguish.

◆   ◆   ◆

March 1986, Tel-Aviv, Israel

Ichilov is a major teaching hospital in Tel-Aviv where I took my post-graduation internship. Part of my education involved training to become an emergency medical services (EMS) physician. In Israel, a physician, usually a "fresh" intern, is required to accompany a special emergency ambulance used for treating very difficult or critical patients. This is called Team-1 EMS[1].

I was one of the four interns participating in a training course to become a physician on Team-1 EMS. All the interns were sitting in a bright small room in Ichilov Hospital. We were listening to a lecture presented by Dr. Bolter, the physician in charge of Team-1. He was an intelligent cardiologist, who had been instructing us on ways to become "rapid thinking physicians" in preparation for dealing with medical emergencies. We were writing notes simultaneously as we intensely listened to him.

"…And the most important thing to offer them is TLC," Dr. Bolter said.

Suddenly, I interrupted his rapid paced lecture with a question.

"What is TLC?" I asked.

"TLC stands for tender, loving care. Don't forget! This is an important part in taking care of a patient," he replied and then moved on to the next subject.

"…If you have any difficulties in managing any patient you should send him or her to the hospital. If the patient doesn't want to be transferred, just get consent. Whenever you don't know something, just ask the paramedic or the driver

---

1.   Team-1 emergency medical services stands for the Hebrew name of urgent medical services for patients or *Shakhal*.

of EMS. They have a lot of experience. They can be a good source of information on any aspect. You just try to take care of the patient; *the rest is up to them.*"

I was a fresh intern, recently graduated from medical school, going through my first month of rotation in cardiology. I was inexperienced about how to handle most unexpected medical situations. I felt I would obtain a solid base of information related emergencies after the rotation in cardiology and the EMS training. In addition, I had the opportunity to rely on many other support sources around me, such as the residents, the attendings, other interns, the nurses, the paramedics, and even the driver of the EMS! No matter what, I was scared! I knew I would be on call alone on many nights. I was aware there would be occasions requiring me to make difficult decisions—hopefully the right ones—all on my own. I felt like going through the internship was an expedition into a dark tunnel while holding a small candle to brighten the path. Only experience would make the candle brighter to see the pathway better.

April 1986, Tel-Aviv, Israel

To be the EMS Team-1 physician was one of the most exciting and demanding experiences that any new doctor could imagine. Early in April, the second month of my internship, I received my call schedule for Team-1. The general rule of the squad was to deliver emergency medical services at the scene. If necessary, we would then transfer the patient to the *nearest* designated hospital. I had reviewed my notes from Dr. Bolter, over and over, hoping to prevent any mistakes. I was fully ready to go, I thought. I felt fortunate to begin this challenge early in my internship. I imagined that an early exposure to unexpected emergencies would make me gain experience faster. Now, I wonder if this was a true perception!

It was a beautiful sunny morning. I had obtained the directions to the EMS building from the medical staff department at Ichilov Hospital. It took me a while to find the building. Upon entering the lobby, across from the entrance, behind a glass wall, a secretary was talking to another person. I hesitatingly interrupted their conversation. "I am the new intern for Team-1. What should I do?" The secretary pointed to the first room on the left down the hall. "That will be your room. You can wait there. We will call you when there is an emergency." Then, she turned her head and continued her conversation with her friend.

I picked up my backpack and went to "my room." It was dimly lit, with one small window overlooking the street. A narrow bed was located in one corner. I placed my bag on the floor and sat down on the bed. Then, I noticed a small closet. All of the sudden, a man entered the room and hung his jacket in the closet. He looked at me for a brief moment, and then said "Hi". I answered "Hi", and then he left the room. Soon, I heard voices of some people talking outside of the room. To satisfy my curiosity of who they were, I walked into the hallway. Several young Israelis were talking about the basketball game from the previous night. I walked up to them and introduced myself. They glanced at me for a few seconds, and then surprisingly, continued talking without any response to my presence. Their behavior appeared strange to me. I did not wish to make any more connection with them, so I returned to my room. It did not take long before a young Israeli man, in his mid-twenties, opened the door and stuck his head into the room. "Hi. I'm Gabby. Are you the doctor?" the man asked. "Yes, I'm the doctor", I answered. "OK, I am the paramedic. Whenever we have an emergency we'll let you know". He closed the door and was gone.

Everyone, from the secretary to the paramedic, had a strange cold behavior. None of them spoke very much. They gave me the feeling that I was nonexistent. Apparently, I was just an extra "item" that was forced on them. Their odd behavior made me extremely nervous and uncomfortable.

While I waited, I opened my EMS notebook to review Dr. Bolter's notes. I was half way through the review when suddenly I heard the speaker announcing "Emergency, Team-1, emergency Team-1." I quickly closed my notebook and returned it to my bag. Swiftly, Gabby entered the room. He opened the closet, picked up his lab coat and said: "Hurry up, let's go!" It did not take long before we were all in the ambulance. Once I was seated in the back, I recognized the driver. He was one of the people who had been talking about the basketball game. When we started to move, I asked, "Gabby, do you know what the problem is?"

"A man fell from a ladder."

"Do we know about the patient's condition?"

"No. We'll find out when we get there", he answered firmly.

The sound of the ambulance siren interrupted our conversation. This was my first mission. My heart was pounding and I could feel butterflies in my stomach. In just a few minutes, we reached the scene of the accident. As my small group approached, I saw an Arab construction worker lying on the ground. From the position of his body and his moaning, we could tell he was in pain. The right sleeve of his shirt was bloody. The ambulance driver carried a very large medication box. Gabby and I started to work on the man.

"Do you want IV fluid? Yes?" Gabby asked. I did not know whether he was asking a question or letting me know what we had to do.

"Yes! Of course! IV fluid is a good choice." I replied with certainty.

Gabby opened the medical box and grabbed a bottle of intravenous fluid, which he prepared for infusion. In seconds, he inserted the IV-lock and started the infusion. I was just watching him. Then, he stabilized the possible open fracture of the man's arm. Everything came to him naturally. I started to write my notes on the patient's paper work. We all helped to lift the man into the ambulance. I sat in the back seat next to the patient. I was pondering who the boss was in Team-1, the doctor or the paramedic!

After we brought the man to the nearest hospital, we headed back to the EMS-building. Gabby and the driver were talking. Again, I had the feeling of isolation. Gradually, I began to realize that Team-1 was made up of three people. One of them changed very frequently. That person was the doctor. The permanent actors in the game were the paramedic and the driver. I sensed that it would be difficult for them to bond with an "outsider" so quickly.

Once the driver had parked outside of the EMS-building, in order to recharge the ambulance batteries, he used a long set of electric cables to connect the ambulance to an electrical socket in the wall. Gabby and I went back to the building. I entered "my room", which, by now, I realized was the room for workers of Team-1. I opened my notebook and restarted my review. Less than 10 minutes later, Gabby opened the door quietly and said, "Dr. Bolter called". He asked us to go and see a patient in her private apartment. She has shortness of breath. Apparently, she is a cardiac patient who has had numerous hospitalizations.

By now, it was 10:00 o'clock in the morning. All three members of Team-1 got into the ambulance again. We drove along a couple of small streets in the heart of Tel-Aviv. Finally, the driver slowed down to find the address. It was a four-story apartment building. In Tel-Aviv, not many small buildings have elevators, but as we entered the lobby, we noticed that one did. This indicated the economic status of the tenants.

At the apartment, a heavy set tall man opened the door. He introduced himself as the patient's nephew. The man directed us inside. I noticed it was a very nice, big apartment.

"Who is the doctor?" the man asked.

"I am," I answered.

"This way please," he said, and led us to his aunt's room. The rays of the sun coming from the window made it delightful.

The patient, an old woman in her late 80's, was lying comfortably in her bed. I approached her. Once she saw me, she half-raised from the bed. She grabbed my hand and began kissing it. That was the first time someone acted this way toward me. I asked myself, "Am I such an important person to her that she has to kiss my hand?" Apparently, I was.

The patient's nephew stood behind me near the window. I sat down on the bed next to the patient and began asking several questions to determine her problem. Meanwhile, Gabby and the driver were trying to hook her up to the ECG machine to trace her heart rhythm. Due to time restraints, many procedures were done simultaneously. While Gabby took the ECG, I reviewed her medications. She was consuming more than ten different prescription medications. Then, I examined her. She appeared very anxious, but without any apparent difficulty breathing. This was contrary to what had been reported to us. Her lung exam was also unremarkable. Her ECG showed sinus tachycardia—a rapid heart rate—and an old heart attack. Otherwise, her exam was unremarkable. After I finished, I held her hand very gently and looked into her eyes. I was trying to comfort her with TLC!

"When was the last time she was in the hospital?" I asked the nephew.

"Ah. This is the story of her life now," he said with frustration. "She goes in and out of the hospital almost twice a month. Just in the last year, she has been in the hospital eight times. The last time was twenty days ago."

This was the first time I would be medically managing a patient without direct supervision. To identify the elderly woman's problem was not a clear-cut diagnosis for me, but I had to make a decision. I remembered Dr. Bolter's phrase, "If you are not sure about your decision, you had better transfer the patient to the hospital." This sounded like a wise decision to me.

"Sir, I don't know exactly why she has shortness of breath. It seems to me that she is suffering from anxiety. Patients with heart disease also may become very anxious," I said.

"So, what do you do for anxiety?" the man asked.

"The only medication that I have in our medication box is Valium. However, I believe we have to transfer her to the hospital."

"OK," the man said. "Transfer her to Ichilov."

Now, it was Gabby's turn to run the show. "We can't transfer her to Ichilov. She has to go to today's designated hospital," Gabby said.

"What do you mean by designated hospital?" the man asked.

"Everyday we take the patients to a different hospital to prevent congestion in the emergency rooms," Gabby said. "Today, Ichilov is not the designated one."

"Oh boy. I am too busy to argue about this transfer. I have an appointment at 12:00 o'clock with Mr. Ariel Sharon, the minister of defense," the man explained.

"I understand how busy you are. However, she needs to be transferred to the hospital," I said.

"OK, if you want to transfer her, you have to take her to Ichilov Hospital," he argued.

"Sir, I can't transport her to Ichilov. We have regulations. I have to take her to the nearest designated hospital," I replied.

"You know what? It doesn't matter. I will take care of it. I will take her to Ichilov Hospital if I have to do so."

"Sir, are you sure about what you want to do?" I asked.

"Yes. I'll take the responsibility," he answered firmly. "Just do something to calm her down".

Before I could reply, Gabby handed me a tablet of Valium.

Shortly after, Gabby ripped a pink paper from our medical progress notebook and left it on the bed. I did not ask what the paper was. I assumed it was the consent form, which we had to leave for the man. Quickly, Gabby and the driver left the room. I felt uncomfortable without my supportive crew. I did not know what else I had to do. I turned around and asked the man one more time, "Are you sure that you can take care of her?"

"Yes. Don't worry about it. If it is necessary, I will take her to the hospital," the man answered.

I left the Valium tablet on the table next to the elderly lady. After looking around one more time, I made my exit.

On the way back to the base, I was emotionally charged about my decisions and wondering about the event. "Was it right to give her Valium? Was her diagnosis really anxiety? Why didn't the nephew want his aunt transferred to the hospital that we recommended? Was he tired of her being hospitalized every third week? Did the nephew know what he was doing? Probably he did! After all, he was an important person, who had an appointment with the defense minister. Should Gabby have done anything else with the consent form?"

I kept thinking about the woman until we reached the EMS building. Team-1 had two or three more calls throughout the day. In all of the cases, we just transferred all of patients to the designated hospital. I had a feeling of satisfaction. I was seeing the real world of medicine, making decisions and carrying them out. I felt joy in being a "real doctor." For so many years, this was what I was longing for. I thought my day was going to end with the most enjoyable feelings.

Around 4:30 PM, half an hour before I would finish my shift, while I was reading a medical book, the secretary knocked on the door, "You have a call from the Ichilov ER-physician. I'll transfer it to your room". In a few seconds, the telephone in my room rang. I picked up the receiver and said "Hello."

"Are you the EMS doctor?" the man asked compellingly.

"Yes, I am," I answered smoothly.

"Did you see an 87 year old lady, complaining of shortness of breath, at her home this morning?" he yelled at me.

"Yes," I answered, hesitantly.

"I want you to know that the family members brought her into the hospital a while ago," he raised his voice more, "Now, she's dead!"

A cold sweat covered me. I remained riveted to my chair. My fingers became numb and the phone receiver almost fell from of my hand. "But the nephew didn't want us to transfer her to the hospital! He gave us his consent!" I said.

"Consent! Where is the consent? I don't see any consent. I don't see any signature. The woman is dead! Do you understand? She is dead...!" He yelled. Abruptly, he hung up the phone.

I was confused. My most enjoyable moment of being a doctor had turned into a dark one. Feeling unable to move, I remained sitting on the edge of the bed. My mind was racing. "Had I really done something wrong? Was the paramedic supposed to get the signature? What was the pink paper that Gabby left on the patient's bed? Wasn't it the consent form? Was I supposed to do the medical part while the paramedic did the rest? What did the patient die from anyway?"

As I was thinking about the incident, Gabby entered the room. I abruptly asked him, "Gabby, did you get a consent from the nephew of the elderly woman we saw this morning?"

"Consent! No. As part of the routine, you were supposed to ask him to sign your progress notes because he rejected his aunt's transfer to the hospital by our ambulance. Did you do that?" he asked.

For the first time someone was telling me "how" to get consent from a patient. "No, I didn't ask him to sign. I thought you did that by leaving the pink form on the patient's bed."

"The pink form!" he said with a smile. "This was just a report of our visit. That doesn't have anything to do with the consent. But, don't worry about it. If there's a problem, we will talk to Dr. Bolter," he said.

"A problem! There is already a problem. The patient is dead!" I said with frustration.

"Oops! That is a problem!" Gabby's eyes opened wide. "Did the nephew complain"?

"I don't know. I am going to find out."

"OK, I'm sorry about that. Anyway, I have to go. You can leave, too. It is 5:00 PM," Gabby said, as he left the room.

I put my book in the backpack and soon left the building. I was eager to discover more about the incident. Therefore, I drove to Ichilov Hospital. On the way, thoughts of being accused by the ER-physician for the death of an elderly woman raced through my mind. When I arrived at the emergency room, the nurses looked at me strangely. It was obvious that the ER-physician's story about a new doctor and the absence of a signature for consent had made quite an impressioin. In the eyes of the staff, it appeared that I was the person responsible for the destiny of "the old lady".

"How did she look when she was brought in?" I asked one of the nurses.

"Oh, it was terrible. She was brought in by her nephew. They came in a private car around 4:00 PM. She was unconscious. She had a whitish foam coming from her mouth. We tried to rescusitate her, but our efforts were futile," the nurse said sadly.

"Did the nephew say anything when she died?"

"Oh, no. He was very understanding about it. He accepted her death very well."

"You mean, he said nothing at all!"

"No, nothing at all," she said.

The nurse's story confused me. I was frightened about the possibility of a malpractice suit against me. Many thoughts surged through my mind. Imagine, a patient had not been transferred to the hospital based on an oral report only, without a written consent. This was the best set up for a medico-legal suit! "Was my diagnosis of simple anxiety correct? Did she have a more complex problem that I, a fresh intern, had missed?" I asked myself. On the other hand, I wondered why the nephew had brought his aunt to the emergency room so late! "Did his meeting with the defense minister have anything to do with it? Upon his return to the apartment, had he found his aunt unconscious? Did the nephew have some remorseful feelings about the death of his aunt? Why was he so calm? Considering his close ties to the government, was he going to persue a malpractice suit against me?"

That night was one of the most restless nights of my life. It was hard for me to fall asleep. I blamed myself for a faulty decision which ended in the death of an elderly woman. The non-stop thoughts of "remorse" occupied my mind. I wanted to be in Team-1 to become a *"real"* doctor, the one who makes decions on his own. This fact indeed happened. However, I was a "real *guilty"* doctor as a result of circumstances. "How could I forgive myself?" I reviewed my action for receiving an oral consent versus the nephew's role—the guarantor's decision—to keep the patient at home. I questioned if my overall assesment and conclusion were the right ones! My subjective thoughts and comments could not change the fact that "my first real patient" had passed away!

I saw Dr. Bolter first thing in the morning. I was anxious to tell him my version of the incident. After I explained what had happened, he shrugged his shoulders and said, "Don't be worried. If there is going to be a claim against you, we will take care of it." He was a source of comfort to me. However, for several days, I was uneasy. Not knowing if any lawsuit action would be claimed against me was troubling. Anyway, I was guilty at least in the eyes of the ER-physician, who scrutinized me heavily because of the death of my first patient.

In the subsequent months, there was nothing heared about the case. I truly believed that the nephew understood the consequences of his decision. Whether he had any feelings of remorse, or not, is the question that I continue to ask myself even until today. Neither he, nor I, knew about the consequences of our actions. However, I had a growing feeling of culpability due to the fact that I was the last physician the old lady saw in her life-time The remorse never left me.

The sense of shame was with me all through my internship and for the next three years in the military in Israel. In the coming years, a deep feeling of condemnation embraced my heart. I felt it every day of my life, from dawn to dusk. Although the uncomfortable sense of remorse did not incapacitate me regarding the making decisions about other patients under my care, nevertheless, it interrupted my rationalizing processes at times. Though difficult, I had to learn how to live with it.

Fall 1992, Hartford, Connecticut

After spending more than three years in military service, residency showed me a different prespective of life. I was fortunate to be accepted into a residency programs which was supported by the best team of teaching physicians. To be a resident is an exciting period for any physician. New challenges are mingled with new ideas. One of the most stimulating occurances that I experienced during my residency program was the weekly teaching grand rounds, which were held by the residents and attendings. It was during one of the grand rounds that I finally found a healing solution for one of the darkest and most painful memories of my life.

Miles away from Israel, as a third year resident in Hartford, Conneticut, I found myself listening to a grand round presented by a fellow second-year resident named Andrea. She was an energetic, intelligent, self confident young woman. I never expected that she would be able to teach each of us a very good lesson. The topic of her discussion was "How do you handle your guilt?". Andrea had such a jovial character that I never imagined she could have feelings of guilt. However, during her presentation, she showed us a completely different picture of herself.

I was sitting in the third row of cushion metal chair in the big auditorium. For about half an hour, I listened to her story concerning her feelings of guilt regarding a medical situation that she had handled. While listening to Andrea, the memories of "my first old lady patient" were renewed in my mind. The years that had passed only made the guilt heavier. This was the first time that I realized someone else had had the same feelings as my own. I began to experience some relief. However, what happened next during the session was to have a dramatic effect on my perspective about what I had gone through all those years.

"Well, I don't believe that I am the only person capable of having feelings of guilt in practicing medicine," Andrea said in her speech. "I would like to ask members of audience to raise their hands if they have had similar feelings". I was shocked by her question. "Do I have to raise my hand?" I asked myself. "What might other people think of me, or about my medical decisions of the past or for the future and…"? Before I could cease my thoughts, I felt my hand rise up into the air. Deep inside, I believed I would have a sense of reprieve from the feeling of guilt I had carried for so many years. Suddenly, I noticed that all the physicians and attendings in front of me raised their hands, too. Since I was on the third row, I turned my head and saw that every one, except two, had their hands raised! It was the most surprising picture that I could ever imagine. I counted forty-two physicians in the auditorium. Almost all of them had experienced some sort of feelings of culpability during their practicing medicine.

The chairman of our department, who had been sitting in the front row, raised his hand as well. Andrea turned and asked him to tell us his story. Our chairman, a man in his fifties, spoke with a very soft tone of voice. His speech was like poetry, full of feelings and experiences. During this time he revealed to us a dark part of his past. He told us his heartbreaking story. One could hardly hear his voice, because it was very dramatic and emotional, as he unfolded his story. Many years ago, when he was an intern, he misdiagnosed a child with meningitis. The child, while under his care, died. Since then, he carried with him the feeling that he was responsible for the death of that child. It was clear, during all these years he had difficulty finding any source of comfort for his pain. Apparently many other physicians in that room experienced the same troubling problems.

After our chairman ended his story, a deep silence came over the audience. This heavy atmosphere expressed a great deal of meaning. No one raised his hand to make any comments or ask any questions. For me, and probably for others, it was a moment of prayer to be better physicians, with or without a sense of guilt. I believe a majority of the audience members shared a very similar feeling at that moment. Obviously, Andrea sensed that we would reach this crucial moment. She dimmed the lights of the room to create a more softening and comforting atmosphere. "Now, I would like to light a candle as a symbol, to relieve all the heavy feelings that we may carry for so many years," she said. "This is for me and each one of us." Then, she lit the candle. We looked in silence at the glowing candle. Some people bowed their heads, probably thinking about what they did in the past.

When the grand round was over, I felt changed. For a longer time than I could recall, I had not experienced this comforting feeling. I realized that my problem was not an isolated one. For some reason, although the sense of remorse was still in place, I had been feeling differently. I felt that I was now a physician with an improved capabilities.

Words can not express fully the impact of that grand round on me. It was not only the most calming lesson that I experienced in my medical career, but also it gave me more strenght to continue with my life. Many years ago, by joining Team-1, I wanted to be a "real" physician. However, the lesson in ethics that I received from Andrea completed the cycle for me to realize its meaning.

Physicians are involved in providing medical care for many patients. They, especially at the early stage of their practices, might be falsely accused of wrongdoing. Some may even do real mistakes, as well as alleged ones. These doctors might self-impose feelings of guilt. I learned during the process of treating patients that once you perform your duties to the best of abilities, you must avoid any sense of remorse over the outcome.

The families and friends of the patients may appreciate a physician for his or her devotion and empathy, but not necessarily because of the knowledge. This is called the "art of medicine". The "real physician" is one who can combine both the art and the knowledge of medicine and use them with the highest accuracy. Other physicians and I have learned this task in much the same way. We had to experience many emotions, including but not limited to guilt, to understand many aspects of human nature.

Some of the names that have been used in this chapter are real names. Mr. Ariel Sharon has been elected as the prime minister of Israel in the year 2000.

MEDICOLEGAL WISDOM

Patients have a right to know about any procedure or treatment, which is ordered for them[1]. **Informed consent** is such information that includes the risks, the benefits, the alternatives and the consequences involved in that medical care.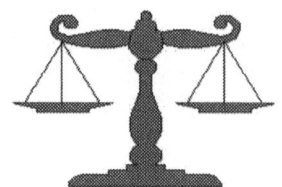

Consents may be given in two forms, oral or written. *Oral* consent, if proved, is as binding as written consent. Generally, there is no legal requirement that a patient's consent must be in writing. However, an oral consent is commonly more difficult to substantiate. *Written* consent has the advantages of visible proof of a patient's wishes and evidence of informed permission.

Consent from the patient is usually required before treatment is begun. However, in routine cases, when an adult patient lacks the capacity of making decisions, consent must be obtained from another person (health care proxy agent), who is empowered to act on the patient's behalf. The agent must receive sufficient information about the planned treatment in order to make a decision consistent with the patient's prior known wishes.

Adult patients who are conscious and mentally competent, or the health care agents of incompetent patients, have the right to refuse medical care that would be considered vital. Noteworthy, patients not only can decline treatment but also may refuse the touching of any part of their bodies by others. Once a refusal of medical care is established, it must be honored regardless of its basis, whether religious beliefs or a mere whim. A legal action for assault and battery might be taken if this right is not respected. In cases of rejection of medical care, every effort, free of threat, should be made to explain the importance of the procedure. Health care professionals are encouraged to pursue the reasons of refusal since they may uncover critical information that may help the patients in their management. The importance of such discovery will be further elucidated in chapter 9.

Shortness of breath (dyspnea)—this is divided Into two essential categories, acute or chronic[2].

Acute shortness of breath may be divide into three subcategories, pulmonary (attributed to lungs), nonpulmonary, and neuropsychiatric:

1. *pulmonary* diseases include pneumonia, pulmonary embolus (migration of a blood clot to the lungs), spontaneous pneumothorax (puncture of the layer around the lungs), asthma, foreign body aspiration, noncardiac pulmonary edema (including noxious gas inhalation, high altitude pulmonary edema, and neurogenic pulmonary edema), and the adult respiratory syndrome (fat embolization, shock lung).

2. the major *nonpulmonary* cause of acute shortness of breath is cardiogenic pulmonary edema (accumulation of fluid in the lungs).

3. Acute hyperventilation syndrome (panic attack or sever anxiety) is a relatively frequent *neuropsychiatric* cause of dyspnea.

Chronic dyspnea are divided into pulmonary or nonpulmonary diseases:

1. *pulmonary* causes are either chronic obstructive airway diseases such as emphysema, chronic bronchitis and chronic bronchial asthma, or restrictive lung diseases which reduce the capacity of the lungs.

2. *Nonpulmonary* causes are congestive heart failure, anemia (deficiency in the amount of the blood), hyperthyroidism (increased activity in the function of the thyroid gland), upper airway diseases, obesity and neurosis (emotional instability)

Each of these categories and subcategories require different treatments.

◆   ◆   ◆

During the years of my practice, I have become more educated about ethics, morals, and medical laws. It was through this knowledge that I discovered how innocent I was in the handling of "my old lady patient". I learned that obtaining an oral consent for an action, in the presence of two witnesses, was enough to justify my decision in this case. There was no need for a written consent from the nephew, although it was a more desirable choice.

How I feel today regarding my old lady's outcome does not eradicate the many years of my enduring the guilty feelings. I wish her cousin had accepted my Team-1 offer to transfer her to the nearest hospital. However, the inevitable outcome occurred. Even after such a long time, I always wonder what her final diagnosis might have been. It is hard to provide a definite answer to this hypothetical question after so many years and little new information. Now, when I think about it, I presume she most probably passed away from a pulmonary embolism. This could be associated with her symptoms of acute shortness of breath and rapid heart beat. This is a common diagnosis in many elderly non-ambulatory people. Some clinicians might overlook this condition. Today, the rate of discovering a pulmonary embolism has been increased by using improved laboratory tests and better tools, such as spiral CT and ventilation perfusion scans.

Since the standards in the medical field are high, many health professionals may have guilt about an ill-fated outcome. After all, a human being is not perfect. It is a difficult task for one, such as a physician, to make hundreds of different decisions on a daily basis. The important key is to be alert to formulate the best judgment! Accumulation of experience of making many decisions over several years eventually improves the quality of the final results. In the field of saving lives, most decisions are aimed toward comforting and curing patients. Most of these choices are correct. Among them, some might even be considered heroic!

4

A Heroic Act

In 1988, after my internship, I became a physician officer in the Israel Defense Army. Military service in Israel is performed without any significant financial compensation. One of my friends helped me to find a weekend job as a night shift physician in a small hospital, called Laniado, in the town of Natanya. The salary was minimal but enough to keep me going.

One Friday afternoon, I drove to Laniado Hospital for my night shift. When I arrived, the doctor of the day, Alon Markowitz, welcomed me to the unit. I knew him from my clerkship. He was a tall man whom I had never seen smile under his thick mustache. His tone of voice was soft, as if he was in full control. It appeared to me his mind was jammed with medical information. You bet; I envied him for his charm and knowledge.

Alon and I visited all the patients for whom I was responsible. This gave me the opportunity to familiarize myself with their cases before I took over. "Mr. Friedman has pneumonia. He is on IV antibiotics," he said as we were doing the round. "The next one is Mr. Schultz. He came in with an attack of gallstone. He had an emergency cholecystectomy to remove his gall bladder. He is stable now. Let's go to the other room. OK, this poor lady is Mrs. Yakovof. As you see, she is jaundiced and unconscious. She has untreatable pancreatic cancer. She is DNR. So let her go if she dies…" We reviewed every one—all 40 patients for that night.

Around 7 PM after I had finished my dinner, I admitted a patient from the emergency room to my unit. Then, I read through the paper work, which consisted mostly of laboratory results. When that was completed, I had an opportunity to sit down to chat with the nurses. They shared their memories with me, not only about the patients but also about themselves. It was a good chance for all of us to get to know each other. I thought this intimacy would help us to work in harmony. Midnight was usually the time to wrap up all the loose ends and get some rest. This was the routine of every on-call night.

Around 2:00 o'clock in the morning, when I was deeply asleep, the telephone in my on-call room rang. I hardly opened my eyes as I reached for the phone receiver. However, before I picked it up, the ringing stopped. "Wrong number," I thought to myself as I drifted back to sleep. It was not long before I heard knocking on the door. "Eddie, you are a heavy sleeper!" said the lady who opened the door. The hallway light penetrated through the doorway into my dark room. I could make out the silhouette of a thin woman against the bright background.

"Oh, Leha, is that you? What is happening?" I asked.

"Why didn't you answer the phone?" Leha, the night nurse, asked.

"I'm sorry. I tried to pick up the phone, but it stopped ringing."

"We kept ringing and ringing but you didn't answer. I don't blame you. You had a difficult day. Anyway, this doesn't matter. You need to get up now. They just rolled in a patient from the emergency room with shortness of breath. You'd better look at him."

"Hold on. I am coming." I got up and rubbed my face to wake up fully. She waited for me at the door. "Do we know this patient?"

"You don't! But he is well-known on the floor for his readmissions," she explained as we walked down the hall together. "He has lung cancer."

"Did you say lung cancer?"

"Yes. You heard it right."

"Do we have a chest x-ray on him?"

"Yep. It's in the room," she said proudly. "I brought it for you from the emergency room because I thought you might need it."

I smiled at her as a token of appreciation. "Let's go and take a look at him."

"Oh, poor guy, he's in a bad shape," said Leha. "We had to put him in the procedural room because we did not have any more rooms for men. Hopefully, we can switch a couple of beds around in the morning to make a room for him."

The procedural room was large. Several storage cabinets occupied the corners, but there was enough space left to allow doctors to perform any procedure. When Leha and I entered the room, we saw an obese man sitting on the bed. He was breathing rapidly. His face was unshaven, clammy, pale, and very tired looking. Although an oxygen mask was on him, I still could see his bluish lips under a thick mustache. I examined him briefly. I discovered that his heart rate was rapid and his blood pressure was low. He looked dreadful.

"Doctor,…help me…I can't breath…I beg…you…doctor," the man said with difficulty.

"OK. Calm down. I'll do my best," I said passionately. Then, I turned to look for the chest x-ray. I spotted it hanging on an illumination box on the wall. As I approached the x-ray, I discovered that a huge amount of fluid had accumulated around his lungs. I realized he was suffering from a condition called pleural effusion. It was obvious that, to ease his breathing and reduce the amount of fluid, he needed to undergo a procedure called thoracentesis. This was one procedure that I always feared because of its possible complications. Now, I had to perform it!

I experienced a flash back to the time I was a third year medical student in clinical rotation. I remembered overhearing a conversation between two internal medicine residents, Alon Markowitz, the senior resident, and Nina Levi, the junior one. Nina was a short, attractive lady. Her rounded face and soft colored blond hair complimented her green eyes. Her movements were quick and unpredictable, as if the world would end the next moment! When we, the medical students, had to follow her around the hospital, we were not walking, but rather running after her! Her job was to be done without any delay. She certainly appeared to be an almost perfect resident.

Alon and Nina talked about a patient who required thoracentesis because of pleural effusion. The patient needed to have the procedure on the same day and Nina was supposed to perform it. I was just a bystander, a frightened student learning about the procedure and its complications.

"How many times did you miss while you did thoracentesis?" Alon asked Nina.

She momentarily glanced down. Then, she gently pulled her right hand from her white lab coat pocket and showed him three fingers. "Three times!" she said with a smirk on her face. I looked at her. This wasn't the speedy Nina that I knew. Her gesture was in slow motion compared to her routine movement. It was obvious! It was as if the phrase "I feel guilty" was written in red all over her lab coat!

"Woo! Did you really miss three times? Wait a minute, how many times have you done thoracentesis at all?" Alon inquired.

"Almost five," Nina answered.

"Mmm…" Alon said and raised his eyebrows. "In three out of five you caused pneumothorax! I think I'd better come to give you a hand with this one."

Nina agreed by responding to him with a big charming smile.

Pneumothorax is actually the result of the perforation of the lungs. Thus, there would be penetration of air around the tissue of the lungs. This error indeed is a serious complication of thoracentesis, which requires more intensive treatment. I believe Alon thought Nina might cause more problems for the patient by puncturing his lungs instead of penetrating into the fluid around the lungs. Later that same afternoon, two other medical students and I anxiously watched Nina as she performed the thoracentesis. This time, she did not miss! "Good job!" Alon commended her after she successfully completed the procedure. It was clear that experience was an important factor in her achievement. I apathetically said to myself, "Well, this is a job for residents and not for students. I'll never have to do that procedure." What a foolish assumption! That day, I learned the technique of thoracentesis. However, I did not have a chance to practice it. Perhaps, my fears helped me escape from performing this procedure at any time during the following years.

Now, many years later, alone, I had to be courageous enough to help a very sick man with a massive pleural effusion. He was a patient suffering from breathing problems. He required an immediate thoracentesis. Without it, he could suffocate to death. I tried to put aside my overwhelming fears. I needed to help my patient by doing that procedure, even though I had almost no experience in performing it. Every second was valuable.

"Sir, I need to draw some fluid from your back to help you breathe easier. Is that OK?" I asked the man.

"Is this...g...going to be...difficult...?" he asked with a great deal of hesitancy.

"I don't believe that the procedure will put you in any more difficulty than you are in now."

"Doctor...just do...whatever you...think is...nec...necessary! Do it...quick!"

While the man was sitting in an upright position, I carefully checked him with percussion and listened to his lungs. I located the precise spot on his back to insert the needle for thoracentesis. First, I cleaned the area with a sterilizing solution. Then, I put on the sterile gloves. Leha handed me a long, IV-lock, which I connected to a syringe. I gently pulled off the plastic sheath of the IV-lock to expose the needle. My breath was trapped in my chest and I could feel my rapid heart pounding! Time seemed precious! I hesitantly stared at the needle. "Just do the right job little fellow!" I said, "I don't want you to cause any problem. And, no pneumothorax!"

I placed the needle against the skin. I felt flushed as I gently pushed it into my patient's flesh. I slightly pulled back the knob of the syringe but no fluid appeared in the cylinder. A cold sweat covered my face and my hands started shaking! Leha was hesitantly looking at me. To bring some confidence to the atmosphere, I asked the patient. "Sir, are you OK?" "Yaa...I am OK," the man answered with a deep voice. I decided to push the needle in a few more millimeters. Still, no luck! "Damn! What a business am I in? Life and death?" I argued with myself, "I have to do what I have to do. I am responsible toward this patient. Be brave! I bet you're in the right spot. But, where is the fluid? Push this needle in until you see the fluid." So I did. I gently advanced the long needle into the back of the man. I pulled back the knob of the needle again. Suddenly, in the dark of the night, I saw the light of hope! A yellowish fluid began to fill the syringe. I took a deep sigh of relief and cheerfully said, "Success!"

"Doc…did you ask me…a question?" the man inquired.

"No, everything is under control!"

"Oh…that's good," he said. He did not know what I had been going through, or how happy I was.

I disjointed the syringe in order to advance the short plastic tube that covered the needle into the back of the patient's chest. Leha connected the tube to a long hose, which was attached to a special jar. Almost a liter and a half of fluid was collected in the bottle before the man began to breathe comfortably. We kept the oxygen mask on him at all times. His gray lips gradually changed to a pinkish color and his breathing slowed down. The time was around 3:30 in the morning. There was no one around to praise me with "Good job" as Alon had done to Nina. I knew, however, that I had performed a heroic deed to save a patient, or, at least, to relieve the man's agony. "Thank you, doctor," the man fluently said. "I feel much better. I can breathe much easier. Thank you, again."

◆   ◆   ◆

During the following days, I could not stop thinking about my performance of that thoracentesis procedure. I experienced a sense of pleasure and a feeling of pride about helping someone at a crucial moment. Many years later, I tried to put my feelings into perspective. I asked myself if, indeed, my act was a heroic one or just a routine treatment. I believe it depends upon how you look at it. A hero is a person who endangers himself to help another human being in an extraordinary fashion. The fact is physicians perform heroic acts every day, either by opening a patient's chest to do a heart surgery or operating on someone's head to remove a tumor. Even a simple act, for example, such as writing a prescription for antibiotics, can be considered a heroic act in the on going war between the human being and microorganisms. In this case, however, the unnecessary use of an antibiotic for a medical condition puts mankind at risk of losing the battle because of the possible emergence of resistant bacteria.

Most of the medical managements can be considered a heroic deed because physicians are in charge of the well-being of patients. This professional group is in the position to help another human being by taking risks at different levels.

However, since society is so accustomed to these acts, they are often considered routine procedures. Society expects that every medical decision should be safe and without any pitfalls. In other words, a physician is expected to be the perfect hero!

Still, as that young physician, I believed, at 2:00 o'clock in the morning on that day, I had performed an extraordinary act to the best of my ability. I was able to help a severely ill patient who was suffering from agonizing shortness of breath. However, the treatment I used would be considered routine for a well-experienced pulmonologist. It all depends upon how we look at the picture.

Physicians help to prolong people's lives for any period of time. For end stage patients, this period might be just days or weeks. It is essential to identify those patients and keep them comfortable during that phase. I suppose I fulfilled my goal for that particular patient at his time of need.

MEDICAL WISDOM

The way that lungs are set is similar to an inflated balloon being placed inside another inflated one (figure 1). The potential space, which is between the two layers that cover the lungs, is called pleural space. A **pleural effusion** (figure 2) is an accumulation of fluid in this space. It is not a disease entity but signals the effect of pleural or systemic disease on the normal daily passage of fluid through the pleural space[3]. The disturbance in this process may lead to formation of extra fluid in that space. Depending on the composition of the fluid, it has different categories. For example, a pleural effusion that becomes infected is called *empyema.* The presence of malignant cells in this fluid may signal the presence of cancer. The discovery and analysis of a pleural effusion provides an opportunity for the clinician to verify the disease, mechanism, or the drug that has caused the effusion[4].

Thoracentesis, the procedure to drain the fluid, can be either diagnostic or therapeutic. Administration of medications, such as sedatives, is usually not necessary prior to thoracentesis. The selection of the site to puncture for the procedure is crucial to prevent complications and obtaining a successful outcome. The patient is examined in an upright position, and then the needle should be inserted below the upper level of the fluid, in the space between the two ribs. **Pneumothorax**, which is penetration of the either lungs and trapping of the air around them as a result of the their puncture, is the most common clinically important complication during the insertion of the needle. However, bleeding, empyema, and puncture of the spleen or the liver may also happen as other problems of thoracentesis. In today's technology, ultrasound may reduce the risk of complications by visualizing the pleural effusion.

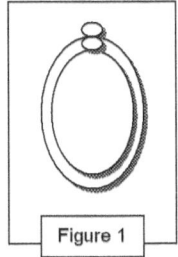
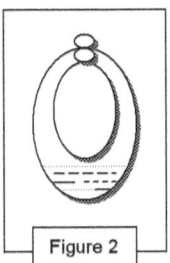

Schematic presentation of normal lungs (figure 1) and pleural effusion (figure 2)

In some cases, the fluid reaccumulates after therapeutic aspiration of the effusion until the underlying condition is improved. An enormous amount of fluid may cause symptoms such as shortness of breath. The effusion in malignancy is usually massive and symptomatic with a high failure rate after thoracentesis due to reaccumulation of fluid[3]. At present, the standard therapy to prevent reaccumulation of the fluid is *pleurodesis*. This procedure creates an inflammatory fusion between the two layers of pleura to eliminate the potential pleural space. These days, physicians may use talc as the preferred agent to cause the inflammation and the subsequent fusion.

◆   ◆   ◆

The memories of that on-call night at Laniado hospital in Natanya have been deeply embedded in my mind. For the entire week after my thoracentesis procedure on that patient with pleural effusion, I was eager to return to the hospital and visit him. The next week, when I was on-call, I arrived on the unit and immediately saw Leha. It made me happy to see her because we had shared "the adventure". Anxiously, I asked her about "our" mutual patient. She said, with sorrow, "He just passed away yesterday due to the other complications of his cancer." I became numb from the shocking news. With a heavy heart, I sat down on the nearest chair. You cannot imagine my immense frustration and dreadful feelings after hearing that news. I leaned my head against the wall and closed my eyes. It was a moment to learn a new reality. I was glad that I was able to relieve that patient's suffering and improved the quality of his last week of life. However, I was a young physician who still had not grasped the idea of the mortality of sick patients.

Cancer and its complications took a patient's life despite the best medical management of that time. Yet, today, this terrible disease may take many lives even with the highest quality of treatment. We, as physicians, still have a long way to go in the battle against cancer.

5

Painful Lesson of Smoking

__Section 1__

It was a year since I established my own medical practice in New York. Now, after many years of different experiences, I had much more self-confidence to make decisions. The office was running smoothly. Every day, I had a fresh adventure to know new people or simply took care of the former patients.

One day, as I glanced at the schedule, I saw a name, James Parlow "Who was this guy? I bet I had seen his name somewhere. Do I know him?" I wondered. An hour later, James arrived at my office. This day marked the beginning of my journey with him.

James, 67 years old, was of Irish descent. His white hair made a nice contrast with his pinkish face. He was tall, but this fact could not mask his round ample size abdomen. James came in because he was experiencing shortness of breath. His initial remark was a quick answer to my inquiry about his well-being.

"Doctor, it took a while before I found you," he said. "I know you from your previous office. You were good. So I came back."

It is always nice to hear compliments from your patients. Nevertheless, the best satisfaction is when you see them alive and healthy. Anyway, I did not leave him without an answer, "James, it is good to see you, too! Probably, it was hard to find me."

"Well, you never forget a good doctor!"

"What can I do for you today, James?"

"Doc., I've had this shortness of breath for the last several days. It just doesn't go away."

By asking him a few questions and examining him, I discovered James suffered from emphysema. His condition was deteriorating due to smoking almost a pack of cigarettes a day. I gave him an inhalation treatment to relieve his symptoms. He felt better. At the end of the session, I prescribed a few inhalers for him and asked him to return for follow-up visits.

In the next few months, it was a struggle to make James stop smoking. Thank God, he was willing to strive. Finally, he stopped completely! I was wondering how long this would last. I continued following him on a monthly basis to prevent him from deviating off his new path.

One day, James began discussing a completely new issue. "Doctor, I'm concerned about my wife. She is losing weight. I don't know what's wrong with her!"

"Well, it is hard to make a diagnosis without seeing a patient. Maybe you should bring her in for an evaluation," I suggested.

"I don't know! She doesn't want to see doctors. But, I'll speak to her."

James mentioned the same subject during his next visit. However, It took about 2 months before I saw Madeline Parlow. On a warm summer day in July, she walked into my office along with James. She was a petite, unpretentious woman. Her brownish, curly hair reached to her shoulders, giving her a more youthful appearance. However, her wrinkles could not hide her age. Later, I discovered she was 63 years old. As soon as she entered the exam room, I detected the odor of stale cigarette smoke. The sagging impressions on both sides of her face made it obvious that she was a chain-smoker. Now, I could understand why it was so difficult for James to quit smoking. His companion was a smoker, too.

"Hi, Mrs. Parlow. How are you doing?" I questioned.

"Hi. My husband is worried about me," she said.

"Doctor, she has not seen a physician since she gave birth to our daughter, Rose," said James.

"And how long ago was that?" I asked.

"About 25 years!" he said.

"Wow! That's a long time!" After a brief pause I continued, "Mrs. Parlow, do you feel OK? Any discomfort or pain?"

"I'm fine. I recently lost a couple of pounds. I just don't have enough of an appetite. That's all. But that's OK. I know there is nothing wrong with me," she said.

I was surprised about her ambivalent attitude. I asked many other questions, but none of her answers directed me toward any possible diagnosis for her weight loss or lack of appetite. As I proceeded with my examination, I discovered a large mass in her abdomen. It was about three times the size of a baseball! Immediately, I knew she was suffering from a dangerous illness. I remained calm, but my mind was in search for identifying a possible diagnosis. After the examination, she asked, "Is that it?" I nodded. "Yes, that's all for now," I replied.

After she was dressed, I asked James and Madeline to come to my consultation room to discuss the additional work-up. During our conversation, she positively refused the idea of hospitalization to conduct the further studies. I had no doubts that it was necessary to act as quickly as possible, especially after I learned they were planning to set sail on a cruise in ten days.

I arranged for Madeline to have CAT scans of both the abdomen and the chest on the same day of her visit. As I proceeded with seeing other patients in my office, Madeline, lying on her back, was going through a CAT scan machine in a radiology office. In a matter of a few minutes, the circular machine took several x-rays of her abdomen and chest. In the observatory room, the technician was controlling the process.

"OK, Mrs. Parlow," said the CAT scan technician as he entered the CT room. "You are done. You can come down." Then, he helped her to get off the table. "Oh, you are so easy to help. You are such a tiny person! There are some overweight people who are difficult for me to help getting down from this table."

"Thank you, sir. Once, I was heavier, too," she said and a smirk appeared in the corner of her face. "I'd better keep going. My husband is waiting for me downstairs. You were very kind."

"You're welcome, ma'am."

The technician followed her with his eyes until she stepped out of the CT room. Then he mumbled to himself, "Poor lady!" He had already speculated the diagnosis from the pictures that he took of her.

Two hours after the testing, I received a call from the radiologist who had the report. The news was what I had expected. "Mrs. Parlow has multiple masses in the both lungs and the liver," he said. "It is probably a cancer of the lungs, which spread to the liver. The biggest mass in the liver is 12 cm," he explained. Experiencing a devastated feeling upon hearing that, I wanted to find a solution. I knew it would be difficult, almost impossible, to save her. Later that day, I briefly discussed the report with James when I reached him by phone. I expressed my highest concern. I suggested that Madeline and James come to my office the next day.

To my astonishment, there was a crowd of six people waiting when I arrived at the office the next day. There was Madeline, James, their two sons, Matthew and Robert, and their daughter, Rose, and her fiancée. James and Madeline took seats next to each other as the family members entered my consulting room. All of them were anxious about Madeline. I could not ignore Rose. She was a young lady whom I noticed squeezed her fiancée's hand from time to time. Her blue eyes were begging me to do something as quickly as possible. Robert, the youngest son, remained quiet, as if the sadness of the entire world was in his heart. The amazing phenomenon was, Madeline showed little concern. She was very calm.

I had a melancholy feeling that with this advanced metastatic lung cancer my help would be limited to supportive care. Madeline was calm because instinctively she knew the end of her life was not too far off. She must have suspected this for some time, probably long before she considered seeking medical help. For me, I had come to terms with the fact that she had a terminal condition. I needed to make this family understand this fact!

"Doctor, can I still smoke?" Madeline asked.

I studied her deeply and then replied, "Yes."

"Doctor, what do you think about the cruise?" questioned James.

"A cruise! Are you planning a cruise?"

"We wanted to be together. We thought the best way to do it, would be taking a cruise," James said.

After a brief pause I said, "I don't see any problem if you want to spend some time together. We surely can continue the management right after you come back from your trip."

"What do you think we have to do in the meantime?" asked Rose.

"A consultation with an oncologist might be helpful to clarify some more facts for you," I said.

"So, you think she'll get chemotherapy," asked Rose.

Madeline cut her off and said empathically, "No therapy at all! I want to go on the cruise." Then, she turned to me and said, "I believe I'll see you after my trip."

"That's quite acceptable to me. Meanwhile, I suggest that you see an oncologist before you go on the trip," I said.

"So be it," Madeline said.

Two days later, I received a call from the oncologist. "Dr. Tabib? Hello, This is Dr. Sheldon."

"Dr. Sheldon! Hi. I'm glad to hear your voice."

"Me, too. I'm calling regarding your patient."

"That has to be Mrs. Parlow."

"You are quite right. I just saw her. She is a very nice lady. Unfortunately, she has metastatic lung cancer. Besides, I don't think that much can be done for it. She and her husband want to go on a cruise. I agreed with you. I gave them the OK." Dr. Sheldon's answer did not surprise me. We both knew it was too late to offer her any treatment.

A week later, James and Madeline departed on the ship. They enjoyed the warm Caribbean weather, ate a lot of delicious food, danced together, and enjoyed every moment. They knew that time was very precious. They would not have each other for too long. It was as if they just discovered each other for the first time. Those were definitely treasured and memorable days, even if Madeline was sick.

Two days after their return, Madeline became very ill. I received a call from Rose, "Doctor Tabib, my mom has difficulty breathing. Can we do something to help her?"

"Does she want to be hospitalized?" I asked.

"No! She said that she wants to stay home. No matter what happens, she wishes to remain here."

"OK. Let's try our best to keep her comfortable. Meantime, I will ask the home care agency to provide you with an oxygen supply. This might ease her breathing."

"Do you think you can give her something to keep her comfortable?" she asked with a trembling voice.

"I can prescribe morphine. This might help her to relax. Is this what you wish?"

"Yes! If that helps her to be comfortable, my answer is yes!"

Later that afternoon, a tank of oxygen was delivered to the Parlows' home. In the late evening, I received a call from the visiting nurse. "Doctor, I'm with Mrs. Parlow. She is quite sick. Her blood pressure is low. Her pulse is rapid. She is kind of sleepy, too. However, she sounds extremely uncomfortable. I just gave her 5-mg of morphine per her request. Is there anything else that you want me to do?"

"Well, at this time, that is all. When will you come back to see her?"

"Probably tomorrow morning."

"All right, I will speak to you in the morning."

I never had a chance to speak to the nurse again. Instead, I received a call from James in the morning. My secretary, Barbara, asked me to take the phone call.

"Doctor, this is James. I just wanted to tell you that Madeline passed away."

"Oh, I am so sorry," I said and I slumped down in my chair. "When did it happen?" I inquired.

"Just an hour ago. It was peaceful. She wanted it this way."

"How are you? How are your children handling it?"

"Oh, they are all here. In fact, they all slept here last night. My house is a small one. Some of them slept on the floor. What can I tell you...! She is gone."

"I am deeply sorry about your loss, James. I wish I could have done better for all of you."

"…Well, this is life. Thank you for your support. Thank you very much."

Madeline had not seen a doctor for the last 25 years. When she finally consented to see one, it was too late! This fact made me extremely sad, especially after I became familiar with all of her family members. Why had she not consulted someone earlier? Why did she not quit smoking a long time ago? Another physician or I could have saved her life with an earlier intervention. Sometimes, we, as doctors, may be able to change the course of a disease depending upon when we become involved. In her case, it was too late to save her. She missed many enjoyable adventures in her life. Among them, Rose was engaged and planning to get married. Now, Madeline would not be present to walk with her down the isle. Madeline departed from her family much too early, ending her glorious life because she turned thousands of cigarettes to smoke!

A few days later, I attended Madeline's wake. Being Jewish, this was my first time going to a wake. It was a small ceremony. Madeline looked beautiful with her make-up, resting peacefully in her coffin. I had a chance to see the rest of the Parlows including James' oldest son, Steven, who was a doctor. Steven had driven all the way from Pennsylvania. They were all saddened, but content with what had happened to Madeline. Everyone appreciated my efforts to keep her as comfortable as possible during the last days of her life.

Madeline's death, however, was not the end of this story. Instead, a completely new chapter was opened between the Parlows and me. In the months following the tragedy, the whole family, including James 93 years old aunt, came to my practice as new patients. I was about to begin another journey with this family.

Section 2

During the month of July, the weather was very warm. Dressed in casual clothes, I was sitting behind my desk struggling to prepare myself for recertification with the Board of family practice. This recertification involves sitting for an exam that I am required to take every 6–7 years. It was very difficult to cut back on the office hours and just "study". I told myself preparation for the exam would be a good review of the medical literature. During that "study" time, I came across a question regarding smoking. It read, "Which one of the following cancers is not related to smoking? A) Gastric cancer (cancer of the stomach), B) Cancer of the lungs, C) Cancer of the bladder, or D) Cancer of the colon (large bowel)". The question surprised me. I thought they all were related and caused by smoking.

The answer given in the article was colon cancer. I thought that could not be correct, but I dismissed it from my mind.

After refreshing my memory with all kinds of medical literature, I returned to the usual matters of business. In the following weeks, I saw Rose several times. I established a very good relationship with her. She was a quiet, young woman with discrete goals for her life. She was passionate about human beings and, above all, devoted to her father, James. She wanted to be a nurse.

In September, I saw James in my office for a follow-up concerning his blood pressure. He told me he had started smoking again after the death of his wife. Otherwise, he was tolerating her loss very well. I urged him to stop smoking. He assured me he would be trying. He also confessed that Rose was throwing away his cigarettes! Due to his age, I suggested that he go for a routine colonoscopy. This is a procedure to check the large bowel. He agreed to have the procedure. Therefore, I referred him to Dr. John Reznick, a gastroenterologist.

It was in late October that James made an appointment with Dr. Reznick. James' first visit with him was pleasant. It was all about a handshake, a quick history, an examination, and preparation orders. The last part was the most difficult one. The day before the procedure, James had to visit the restroom so many times because of repeated bowel movements! He was sure he had followed the instructions as recommended. He thought, "I hate this colonoscopy. First, you get diarrhea. Then, the next day, someone puts a tube into your butt! Can't they come up with something easier?"

The day of the colonoscopy, James was extremely nervous. Finally, the moment arrived. After he was comfortable on a table, an anesthesiologist put a mask on his face. Then, they gave him an intravenous injection. He felt very tired right after that. The next thing he realized he was in the recovery room. The procedure was easier than he thought. For James, the "actual pain" was to come much later.

One afternoon in November, I received a very disturbing call while I was in the middle of a conversation with a patient in the exam room. My secretary asked me to answer a phone call from Dr. Reznick. I excused myself to speak with him. I picked up the phone in my private consulting room.

"Hi, Ed, how are you?" he asked. I recognized distress signals in his voice.

"I am fine, John. What's happening?" I asked.

"Listen, do you remember the guy you sent to me for colonoscopy, Mr. Parlow...?"

A squeezing feeling in my chest alarmed me. "Yes, I do. What's up with him?"

"I took out 3 small polyps. I just got the biopsy report. One of them was malignant!"

"Oh, boy!" I said. My heart skipped a beat. I had to sit down to continue the conversation. "Are you sure about it?"

"Yes. Only one is cancerous."

"That's all James needed, cancer of colon." I thought. "Well," I said, "he will probably requires surgery. Does he know about this?"

"No," he said.

"OK, I have to speak to him."

"OK, let me know if I can be of any more help."

It was difficult to believe! First James' wife, and now he, himself, was suffering from the devastating disease of cancer. It seemed like he was standing on the *edge of a cliff* about to fall. I felt I had to do everything in my power to save his life! He was only 68 years old. Knowing that his aunt had reached the age of 93, I believed that he had the potential for a long life. An open question was disturbing me, "What could I attribute to be the cause of his colon cancer?"

I completed the visit for the patient who was waiting in the exam room and returned to my desk. I made a phone call to James. He was not at home. Trying to call Rose was also futile. I left a message at her work. One hour later Rose returned my call. "Dr. Tabib, is everything OK?" she asked.

"Yes. I need to talk to your dad," I answered.

"Oh, dad is with his aunt."

"Good, I will give him a call there."

"Is everything OK? Please, doctor, if there is anything wrong, let me know!" her voice was devastating to me.

"Let me talk to your dad first."

"Dr. Tabib, I sense that something is wrong. But, OK. I'll wait until you talk to my dad."

Rose's words were haunting me, but I had to inform James first. When I located him, our conversation was very brief. I made him alert, but not nervous. "James," I said, "I don't know how to break this news to you, but your biopsy wasn't good. I want to see you tomorrow to discuss your situation."

"OK, doctor, I'll see you tomorrow," said James.

The following day, James came to my office alone. We sat down and I described to him the nature of his disease. I told him that he required surgery. I also explained what he should expect during and after the surgery. He stared at the floor for a moment, and then, as if he woke up from a deep sleep, raised his head and said, "I'll do whatever you suggest."

"For a faster recovery, it is important to stop smoking. Have you stopped smoking?" I asked.

"It's already been two weeks since I quit smoking."

"Very good! This lowers the risks of complications during and after the surgery."

Considering James' medical history of high blood pressure, emphysema, and being a smoker and obese, I was very aggressive about his pre-surgical work-up. Prior experiences taught me that anything could go wrong in such a scenario—a heart attack, a stroke or an infection. He could even die during this surgery. I did not know if his cancer had spread. I felt a high responsibility for his life and did not want to let him fall from the *edge of the cliff*. I could not imagine his children losing both parents in such a short period or having a disabled father after this surgery.

I decided to send James for a special test to evaluate the coronary arteries, which supply blood to the muscle of the heart. The test is called a Thallium stress test. I was not surprised when I received James' stress test report. His scans showed a defect, indicating a possible problem in the musculature of his heart. Time was an important factor. We had to do the surgery as soon as possible to prevent any possible spread of the cancer in his colon. Now, however, I was confronted with the fact that his heart might be in danger. Not only James, but also all of his family, was on full alert again! They were all facing a new challenge in their lives.

I hospitalized James for an angiography to evaluate the arteries of his heart. This time I received a reassuring telephone call from the cardiologist. He told me that James' coronary arteries were fine and the Thallium stress test was misleading. This information gave me a green light to go ahead with the recommended surgery. I felt good! Yet, it was not the time to take a sigh of relief. The cancer was still in James' body.

Ironically, that same day, I heard news on the radio regarding new information concerning colon cancer. A study had come out indicating there was a link between smoking and the development of colon cancer. The circumstances reminded me of the question I had encountered while preparing myself for the board exam six months earlier! No one can predict how much we will come to know. Now, I could blame largely James's cancer on smoking, the very same chemicals which had contributed to the death of his wife Madeline. In addition, genetic factors, being over-weight, and having an inappropriate diet, each one played a part in the development of his cancer.

James was hospitalized awaiting the contemplated surgical removal of his large bowel. Meanwhile, I asked a young but highly experienced surgeon, Dr. John Montgomery, to perform the surgery on him the next day. James required a repeat colonoscopy to evaluate where to have the resection of his large bowel. He became upset upon hearing this news, but he soon felt more assured when we informed him this would be done under general anesthesia immediately before the surgery. With this, I left him in the hands of the surgeon. All I could do was pray for James and his family.

The next day, I went to see James in the hospital. I found him lying on the bed. He was hooked up to different wires and lines. A small nasal tube was giving him oxygen. He was experiencing a great amount of pain for which he was not prepared.

"Doc, every time I breathe it is like being stabbed in the abdomen. But, you know what? Finally, I went through it! But, I sure feel terrible!" he said. Then a smile crept into the corner of his mouth. "Doc, how am I doing?"

"You are doing OK, James". I said. "It takes a while, but you will be fine. Just try to rest."

"What can you do about this pain? Any remedy for it?"

"You will receive more painkillers."

"Once I feel better, just get me out of here!"

"I'll sure do."

As I left him, I was still worried about the possibility that the cancer had spread. I could not reveal any of my fears to him right at that time. Two days later, when I accidentally met Dr. Montgomery in the hallway of the hospital, a smile on his face was the answer. "James was a lucky guy. No metastasis! Everything is negative, including his lymph nodes," he said. I smiled back at Dr. Montgomery. This was the best news of that day! Now, I could breathe a sigh of relief! James had been able to step away from *the edge of the cliff*.

When I informed James and his family about the results of the biopsy, they all were relieved and extremely happy. James was discharged from the hospital in less than a week.

A few days later, I saw him in the office for his post-operative follow up. As I examined him, I discovered the first complication. The site of the incision had become infected. Fortunately, it was not too deep and could be treated with an antibiotic. When I saw him several days later I asked him: "Do you still smoke?"

"No way!" answered James. "It makes me nauseous whenever I think about the pain that I had after the surgery! It is over for me!"

James learned about the devastating effects of smoking the hard way. It would have been possible to avoid all of the pain and complications associated with using cigarettes. Madeline could have lived longer, too.

MEDICAL WISDOM

Tobacco is the only _legal, over the counter, harmful, and addictive chemical_ sold worldwide

---

Nicotine is an addictive medication comparable to heroin. A cigarette contains nicotine, tar, and carcinogenic chemicals. Upon usage, nicotine constricts the blood vessels causing a decrease of nutrition and oxygen to the tissues. 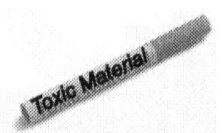 This kind of deprivation, combined with the carcinogens, may easily lead to the development of cancer.

Many different cancers are definitely linked to cigarette smoking. Some of these are throat cancer (laryngeal cancer), which may involve the vocal cords, and cancers of the esophagus, stomach (gastric cancer), lungs, kidneys, bladder, and colon[22]. Lung cancer is the primary leading cause of cancer death in men.

In addition, smoking may cause an increase in the number of the wrinkles on the skin. It may change the environment of the mouth, leading to the development of oral thrush or disrupting the sense of taste. In the throat, it may affect the vocal cords causing hoarseness. In the lungs, smoke can lead to chronic bronchitis and emphysema, which are known as chronic obstructive lung disease in medical literature. After many years, chronic obstructive lung disease may cause a condition known as pulmonary hypertension, which is an increase in the pressure exerted on the arteries exiting the right side of the heart. Deformation of the internal lining of the body's vessels, causing high blood pressure (systemic hypertension) of the body, is another major catastrophe (see chapter 12). These changes in the vascular system of the body may result in heart disease, causing many patients to eventually suffer and die from a heart attack.

The best treatment is prevention. Smoking cessation is not an easy task, but it is possible. A strong desire to stop is necessary. There are chemical agents for help with cessation such as nicotine patch, gum or nasal spray and oral medications, such as Bupropion (Zyban®). Using these aids, in conjunction with behavioral therapy, may lead to successful smoking cessation.

Colon cancer is one of the major causes of death. Not only colon cancer, but also all cancers are the result of changes in the genetic make-up of cells, thus leading to the formation of cancerous cells. A genetic predisposition, such as having one or both parents diagnosed with colon cancer, may amplify the chances of developing this cancer. Some diseases, such as ulcerative colitis, or factors such as, obesity, high fat diet, consumption of more than seven drinks of alcohol per week, and smoking may increase the risk of developing colon cancer. A diet rich in vegetables and natural calcium (probably not calcium in a pill), high fiber diet (such as in cereals), and vitamin D (at least 100 IU a day) may reduce the risk of this cancer. Taking medications, such as non-steroidal anti-inflammatory drugs (e.g., aspirin and ibuprofen) has also shown reduction in development of colon cancer[25]. Obviously, consumption of these medications is not without risks.

Unlike many other cancers, colon cancer is preventable. It can also be curable in early stage. Small polyps in the large intestine may grow to be cancerous. A procedure called colonoscopy may detect these polyps and allow the physician to remove them by using a fiberoptic tube. By removing these growths early, the chances of developing cancer may be reduced to nothing. The colonoscopy is done under mild anesthesia and is generally well tolerated. Performing the initial screening colonoscopy is recommended at the age of 50 years. Depending upon the findings during the initial colonoscopy, and the family history, the gastroenterologist may recommend performing this procedure every 3 to 10 years. The preparation of virtual colonoscopy is similar to routine colonoscopy. However, instead of directly visualizing the inside of the large bowel using a fiberoptic tube, a CT scan takes 3-dimensional pictures to evaluate the internal lining of the colon. Some centers began using a miniaturized camera as another new technique, called capsule endoscopy. It is preferred to identify lesions in the small intestine since the battery-life of the capsule is limited. The patient swallows a smart built-in-digital-camera pill in order to take numerous pictures of the entire intestine. The caveat in the last two techniques is lack of having the ability to perform biopsy. Finding a polyp by any means eventually may require a routine colonoscopy for its removal.

A patient of mine, whose large bowel had been completely removed due to ulcerative colitis, complained of having pain on the left side of his abdomen. When I referred him for a regular x-ray, I incidentally discovered a small screw on the right side of his abdomen. He denied accidentally swallowing any screw. Not knowing what tests he had done in the previous year, I referred him to his regular gastroenterologist. Further investigations were quite intriguing. When the patient heard the news, he laughed. The screw was actually the camera pill that he had swallowed a year earlier for evaluation of his bowel, but it had not left his body! Although uncommon, the capsule may remain in the bowel for an extended period. In this case, there was no connection between that patient's pain and the remnant of the camera-pill.

The earlier signs of colon cancer might be bleeding, abdominal pain, and changes in bowel movements. The treatment for colon cancer is the resection of the part of the large bowel containing the tumor. If the cancer has spread, chemotherapy may be advised.

◆   ◆   ◆

Back to the story...

Two and a half years after her mother's death and right before Christmas, Rose Parlow entered my office for a visit. She carried someone else with her—a three-month old baby girl. A small green and red Irish-style blanket was wrapped around the baby. Her large, wandering, bluish colored eyes met my brownish ones, trying to discover a new person. She giggled and moved her hand exposing her face and her pinkish dress. The combination of her white, soft skin and the colorful clothes made her very attractive. I learned the baby's name by asking Rose during her prenatal care. You can guess the baby's name, too! Her grandmother, if she were alive, would have been proud of little Madeline.

6

Mid-life Challenges

Daniel's first visit to my office was for a physical exam. He was a middle-aged overweight man, with a receding hairline. He was dressed in an elegant black suit with a stylish colorful tie. His shoes were perfectly polished in a manner that reminded me of a marine. We shook hands and he sat down on the chair. He displayed his first charming smile, but I could not dismiss his yellowish teeth and the smell of stale cigarettes that came from his mouth. We chatted for a while. I learned he was the type of man who wanted to know if "he was OK", but did not want to learn how he could "keep himself OK". In other words, he came in to discover if he was in a good state of health, but he did not realize that obesity and smoking two packs of cigarette a day would have harmful effects on every organ of his body.

"You know, you are in good shape. Nevertheless, I recommend that you stop smoking," I said to Daniel when I finished examining him.

"Doc, ask me anything but this! A cigarette is my friend! Forget it! I cannot stop smoking!" Daniel said with defiance. As he was putting on his clothes, I noticed a pack of cigarettes bulging out of the pocket of his jacket.

"I'd better stay quiet," I thought to myself. "He is not ready to quit now. Any comments about his attitude might antagonize him. Then, I would never see him again or have a chance to persuade him to change his unfavorable behavior."

Daniel was not a frequent visitor to my office. His visits were limited to simple medical problems or a general check-up. I was eager to see him slim down and without a pack of cigarette in his pocket. So, during every visit, I reminded him about his diet and his habits. Unfortunately, the answer was always "No". As a matter of fact, I was apprehensive, at times, about discussing any health issues or behavioral modification with him because of his impatient reaction.

My failure to help Daniel's attitude about his health caused me to feel emptiness every time he left my office. As a physician, I was taught, that being able to change any long-standing behavior of a patient might be a prolonged process.

This challenge is often very frustrating for a physician due to the many obstacles along the way. For example, the individual might modify his or her behavior for a short time, and then return to the previous habits. Patience, consistency, close follow-up, and providing a supportive environment are the key elements in the successful process of habit modification.

Daniel was an intelligent, well-mannered person. For years, Daniel politely pushed aside my attempts every time I wanted to discuss the subject of smoking with him. At times, I was even annoyed with his inflexible mind-set. Finally, after seeing him periodically over six years, I asked him exasperatingly, "What has to happen to make you stop smoking?"

"A disaster! I will stop when a disaster happens!" He answered.

Smoking cessation or modifying of one's diet might be very difficult tasks, especially for patients with little desire for changing habits. Daniel's approach seemed to be a self-destructive type of behavior, possibly the result of some depressive elements. Logically, it sounded unintelligent to wait for a disaster to occur in order to change his behavior. What was he waiting for before putting down the cigarettes—Cancer of the lungs, severe bleeding from his stomach, difficulty breathing, or a heart attack?

Finally, during the seventh year of treating Daniel, I received a startling phone call from him. This call brought the first concession after many years of argumentative discussions that I had with him. "Doc, I am on a diet and I am losing weight!" It was shocking news to me to imagine that he actually was informing me, for the first time, about a change in his approach toward life!

"How did you do that?" I asked him.

"I eat less carbohydrates and more meat. Something similar to the Atkins' diet."

"Atkins' diet! But, this is not an acceptable medical diet. The weight loss essentially comes from fluid loss rather than an actual weight loss from fat."

"Doc, you asked me to lower my weight, so I am doing it in my own way! You know what? It is working!" he said firmly but gently enough to avoid any further confrontation.

No matter how persuasive I might be, arguing with Daniel was useless. However, to give him credit for modifying his attitude, I congratulated him on his success as we ended our conversation. I encouraged him to look for other venues for weight loss. Unexpectedly, he showed some flexibility, which was not typical for him.

The notion of "never give up" finally proved itself. After seven years, I could see that, even Daniel, a stubborn patient, eventually might change. His tough

attitude had been carved away by my consistency like a river that eventually pol-
ishes the surfaces of its rocks. However, I considered the modification of his diet
as a small success. As I realized that a behavioral change in a person couldn't happen over night, I had also learned that a big success is based on the accumulation
of small ones.

The changes in Daniel's attitude coincided with his fiftieth birthday. I had a
sense that he knew he was playing with fire. He was not blind to the fact that
being overweight and a smoker might cause many health problems. By the same
token, he was unable to disassociate himself from his troublesome behaviors. He
still wanted to know if he was healthy enough to continue smoking or have an
unacceptable diet.

Daniel's appointment for a physical exam was a few months after his resolu-
tion to reduce his weight. In comparison to his previous visits, Daniel had really
lost a good amount of weight. He was in a good mood and presented himself as a
prosperous businessman. By showing off his success, he intended to convey the
idea that smoking was a harmless act.

"How is everything, Daniel?" I asked.

"Very well. I feel great! Thank God, my business is flourishing and the family
is well! But, you know me. I want to be checked."

"I see that you lost some weight."

"Doc, I told you that I'd do it! Didn't I?"

"Well, it is a good start. But, I am not so sure that you selected the correct
manner to lose the weight."

"Doc, life is about challenges."

"Challenges! Do you know to what topic this conversation may lead?"

A big smile appeared on his face. "I know! I know! You are talking about my
smoking cessation."

"Any hope for the near future?"

"Doc, please! Talk about anything else except this one! You know it is hard to
kick this habit of mine."

I felt that he was still not ready to quit smoking. I concluded our conversation
and proceeded with the physical exam.

"Would you like to step on the scale?" I asked.

"Well, why not."

"Doc," he asked as I was finishing checking his weight, "how much did I lose
since my last visit?"

I compared his current weight with his previous record and I said, "about 15
lbs."

"You see, doc! You just didn't believe me. Guess what? This is only in the last 3 months!"

"Hey, that is good." Then I continued, "Daniel, please understand. With your high protein diet, part of your weight loss is due to fluid loss rather than an actual loss from fat."

"Doc, we'll see. I'm gonna lose even more"

I examined the rest of his body without finding any abnormalities. Then, I said, "Listen, you need an annual rectal exam".

"A rectal exam! Oh sure! Is it necessary doc?"

"Yes, indeed," I answered.

While I was putting on a pair of gloves, I asked him to be prepared for the test. As I was examining him rectally, I palpated a small area of firmness in one of the lobes of his prostate. When I finished, I compared the findings of this exam with the notes from the previous year. I was surprised from the discrepancy between them—new firmness in his prostate!

As I was going through the pages in the chart, Daniel asked, "Doc, is there anything wrong"?

"Daniel, it appears there is something in one of the lobes of your prostate. I did not find this in last year's examination."

"So, what do we have to do?"

"Well, since I did not feel it last year, but I feel it now, it means this is a new finding."

"What do you think it is?" he asked

"Daniel, I don't know yet. I think it is prudent to evaluate your prostate in more detail."

"Do you think it is cancer? You know, my mother had cancer. She died from it. Is this what will happen to me?"

I sensed the anguish in his eyes. I wanted to avoid any definitive answer. "I know about your family history," I said, "What you really need is to see a urologist. You may need some work-up."

He remained silent, momentarily. "Well, whatever you say doc. If this is what you recommend, I'll do it," he said.

At the end of the session, I ordered some blood tests, including PSA. Then, I referred him to a urologist for evaluation. As he left, I felt that I might hear from him very soon.

Daniel's visit with the urologist's office was full of unexpected surprises. Upon entering his waiting area, the small size of the room and the gray color of the walls made Daniel feel disheartened. When his name was called, he felt butterflies in his stomach and a cold sweat covered his face. In the exam room, he patiently waited for the physician.

Dr. Banaroda was a bald short man. The buttons of his long white lab coat could barely close because of his rotund abdomen. After a quick briefing, he began to read Daniel's records.

"Well," Dr. Banaroda said, "I see that your doctor found a nodule in your prostate."

"What did you say? A nod…what?"

"A nodule!" He said, "This is what he found. Don't worry about the medical terms. Evidently, this is a new condition in your prostate. OK, you can get on the table for examination."

Daniel felt confused by the medical terminology the urologist used. However, he did not have any other choices but to follow the doctor's directions. So, as he got on to the table, he turned toward the wall as he was directed. Meanwhile, the doctor prepared himself for the examination. Daniel could not see what he was doing. The doctor remained quiet until he was in the middle of examining Daniel's prostate. Then he said, "Oh! Your family doctor was right! There is something there".

When Dr. Banaroda finished he asked Daniel to put on his clothes and come to his consultation room. As Daniel entered the room, his attention was drawn to the physician's desk. The desk was so completely covered with piles of papers that one could hardly find an empty space. The urologist, who was seated, opened the conversation, "Listen, you need an ultrasound and probably a biopsy of your prostate to find out what's going on there. We can schedule it for next week."

"A biopsy! How do you do a biopsy?"

"Well, first we have to look at your prostate with ultrasound. Then, by using a sort of retractable needle, I take tissue samples from suspicious areas."

"Is this going to be painful?"

"You might feel some discomfort. Hopefully you won't feel much pain."

"Is there anything else that I should know?"

"Yes. Do not take any aspirin."

"I am not on aspirin."

"Oh, all right. So, you just have to take an antibiotic."

"An antibiotic? What is this for?"

"To prevent infection."

The urologist found a small island of empty space in the sea of papers on his desk. He proceeded to write a prescription for an antibiotic. "Take this as I pre-scribed," he said, as he handed the prescription to Daniel.

When Daniel left the urologist's office, he was petrified. "Oh, my gosh! I never imagined I would have to go through this kind of test—a biopsy of my prostate! What if he finds cancer in my prostate? Then, what do I do? I'm only fifty years old! Am I going to survive, or will my life be cut short? I have so many plans that I want to achieve in my life…"

Mentally depressed and agitated, Daniel went to work the next day. He made a few telephone calls to his friends to find out if they had experienced similar problems with their prostates. When he talked to Isaac, his close friend, he learned about the PSA. "It is a blood test for detecting cancer of the prostate. Ask your doctor to do that for you," Isaac said.

"PSA?" Daniel asked. "You mean, by a simple blood test they can determine if I have cancer?"

"It gives them some indications," he said.

Shortly after Daniel's conversation with Isaac, he phoned me to obtain some information about his PSA. "Doc," he asked, "did you check my PSA?"

"Yes, I did. Is there anything wrong?" I asked.

"Doc, I want to know about my PSA. Is it too high?"

"No, it is actually very low,"

"So, this means that I don't have cancer?"

"Well, I can't give you a definitive answer, yet," I explained. "It is correct that the level of PSA may go up with cancer, but you may not see the rise in early stage of the disease. Anyway, you were supposed to see the urologist. Did you see him already?"

"Yes, I did. He scheduled me for a biopsy. Is that dangerous, doc?"

"Well, I'm not surprised about his recommendation for a biopsy. It might be uncomfortable, but if he said so, you'd better go for it."

That same day, when Daniel arrived at home, he sat on his sofa and pulled out a cigarette to smoke. He looked at it and thought, "Are you a friend or a trouble maker"? Then, he slowly rolled the cigarette between his fingers for a while, and eventually lit it.

"Are you hungry?" asked his wife, Sandra, as she entered the room. She wore a black and white dress and appeared well groomed. Her shining eyes were small and her voice was soft.

"No, I am not," Daniel abruptly answered.

"Are you OK?"

"Since when are you interested in how I feel?" he raised his voice.

"You always have an attitude. Does this have anything to do with your doctor's visit two days ago?"

"Now, you want to know about my health. That's very interesting." Daniel said with hostility, while he flicked his cigarette in the ashtray.

"Daniel, what's wrong with you? Is there some problem and you won't tell me? Your behavior has changed in the last two weeks. You know that I'll eventually find out. You'd better tell me now!"

Daniel sat quietly for a while, and then said, "There is something wrong with my prostate!"

"Oh, my gosh! Oh, my gosh!" she said hysterically. "I knew something was wrong! I bet that they found cancer and you aren't telling me. Please! Please! Tell me the truth! I have to know the truth…"

"That is why I don't tell you anything. You get panicky. First of all, they still don't know what's going on. Secondly, don't jump to conclusion."

Daniel did not have a secure marital life. He and Sandra could always find a subject to debate. Through the years of their marriage, instead of supporting each other to resolve their issues, they chose argumentative discussions. His medical problem only added to the on-going tension between them.

A few days later, Daniel had an appointment for the biopsy with his urologist at 3:00 o'clock in the afternoon. He was very nervous. Before noon, he had finished almost an entire pack of cigarettes prior to his new adventure. After a short delay in the waiting room, he was asked to enter the procedure room. A nurse asked him to sign a consent form for the biopsy. He glanced at it briefly and signed it. "Please put the gown on," the nurse requested. He put the gown on and waited. A few minutes later Dr. Banaroda came into the room.

"Hello Daniel. Are you ready? You look anxious. Don't worry about the procedure. I'm sure everything will go well," the doctor said. "Now, you better get on the table and be prepared".

Daniel lay down on the exam table and turned toward the wall. He thought, "I really hope that he will be right and things go well."

"Are you with me?" the doctor said, "I'm going to start."

"Oh, yes," Daniel said. Then, he apprehensively continued, "Please be as gentle as you can. Would you inform me about what you are doing at each step?"

"No problem," the physician said. "Well, first I have to visualize your prostate."

It did not take long before Daniel felt a gradually increasing pressure in his rectum. "What is that?" Daniel asked.

"This is the ultrasound."

Shortly after, Daniel felt a series of pinching-like pains in his rectal area. "Are you done, doctor?" he asked, as he ground his teeth to cope with his discomfort.

"I'm taking the biopsies. Just hold on a few more minutes."

"Here we are. It is done," the doctor said. Subsequently, Daniel felt a relief of pressure in his rectum. It was just a routine test for the urologist, but an inconvenient and uncomfortable one for Daniel. When Daniel got up, the table paper was completely damp from his perspiration.

"OK. We are done," the doctor said. "I hope that it wasn't too bad. The pathology report will be ready in a few days and we can discuss the results at that time."

"Would you be kind enough to submit a copy of the report to my family doctor?"

"No problem."

On the way home, he smoked one cigarette after another. Later that night, a few hours after the biopsy, Daniel was scared to death after he had a bowel movement. "Blood!" he thought and his heart began pounding rapidly. "What the hell! Why am I bleeding? The urologist hadn't said anything about bleeding. What is this? Why is this happening to me? Is this normal? How long am I going to bleed like this? I'd better call the urologist. But, where am I going to find the doctor now, at night?" Then, as he was terrified, he said to himself resolvedly, "Maybe it will stop tomorrow."

Daniel still was bleeding the next morning. Alarmed, he called Dr. Banaroda's office. The secretary answering the phone said, "The doctor is in surgery today. Would you like him to return your call?" Daniel did not have any other choices but to wait. Throughout the day, he experienced intermittent bleeding. The urologist called him back in the evening to give him reassurance that the bleeding could be "normal" and it would stop very soon. However, Daniel kept bleeding. Finally, it stopped after three days.

A few days later, Daniel called my office. He spoke with a trembling voice, "Doc, did you receive the report of my biopsy?"

"Not yet! Is there anything wrong?"

"I don't know. The urologist's secretary told me today that the pathology report is ready, but I have not heard from him yet. May I ask them to fax you the report for your review?"

"Sure! Ask them to fax it over now."

"Doc, you are great! I'll be in touch with you later."

It wasn't long before I heard my fax machine ringing. It was receiving Daniel's pathology report. Like many other diagnostic tools in medicine, a pathology report can fall into a gray zone. So it was with Daniel. The finding was interesting enough to prompt me to place a call to the pathologist to verify its validity.

Daniel called me half an hour after I received the report, "Doc, did you receive the fax? Would you let me know what the urologist found in my prostate?"

"Daniel, I'd better go over your report with the pathologist first before I talk to you."

"Doc, is it so bad?"

"I don't know yet. I promise to call you back."

"Doc, please help me! I'm so nervous!"

"I want you to calm down. Let me do my investigation."

Daniel appeared to be in a panic. He expected an immediate response, which was difficult to grant. I had to buy some time until I could obtain the final comment about his report. I was fortunate to locate the pathologist who read the slides on Daniel's biopsy. He gave me enough information to understand the report and be prepared to explain the subject in simple term to my distressed patient. However, Daniel showed how desperate he really was, because he called me again in less than an hour.

When I picked up the phone, he asked keenly "Doc, what is PIN?"

"How do you know about your diagnosis?" I asked.

"Well," he laughed sarcastically, "I finally found the urologist. He said that I had to repeat the test in 2–4 months. However, he did not go into details. Would you please explain what is going on with me," he inquired. It appeared Daniel needed a second opinion at this point about the future plans for his prostate work-up. "PIN or prostatic intraepithelial neoplasia is considered a precancerous condition," I explained. "It means one step before cancer. The pathologist, to whom I spoke, confirmed the recommendation of your urologist. You indeed may need a repeat biopsy in a few months."

"OK. If that's the case, I'll do whatever you say."

Three days later, Daniel surprisingly came in for an office visit. He appeared pale and the pink color of his lips had almost turned gray. He looked so tired, like a person who had not slept for days.

"Daniel, what is going on? Are you OK?" I asked.

"No! I'm not OK! Doc, there are so many thoughts in my mind. I'm just fifty years old! How can I have a problem in my prostate? This urologist is not very helpful! He sometimes uses medical terminology that I don't understand. Let's forget that his office is a mess and depressing. I was bleeding for three days and he even didn't suggest seeing me. In addition, I don't feel comfortable with him. I think I have to change to a different doctor."

"It's up to you. If you are not comfortable with him, let's find another physician you are contented with."

"I also would like to discuss something else with you."

"OK, I'm listening."

"I'd like to quit smoking!"

"What?" I said excitedly. "Did I hear it right? Do you finally want to quit smoking?"

"Yes, doc! You heard it right. I need some medication to help me do that."

Once, Daniel said he would stop smoking only if a catastrophe occurred. Well, this was his catastrophe. Having a serious condition in his prostate was the catalyst. It is always gratifying for me to see a patient decides to end the use of tobacco. This was the first time Daniel had considered leaving behind one of the biggest habits of his life. The discontinuation of any habit, especially the ones involving addiction, can be very difficult. However, Daniel gave me this time the impression of being prepared for the challenge. I discussed different options of treatment regarding smoking cessation with Daniel. Finally, he agreed to take a medication to help him with the withdrawal symptoms. He was to return for a follow up visit in two weeks. I was enthusiastic to see if his firmness of conviction, combined with medical treatment, eventually would make him smoke free.

Three days later, Daniel left his house early to go to work. As he sat behind the wheel of his car, he recalled having a pack of cigarettes hidden in the glove compartment. He opened the compartment door and found the pack. He pushed a cigarette out, looked at it and put it back. "Not today!" he said. He smiled, relishing the feeling of his will power.

While cruising on the highway, he glanced at the glove compartment one more time, but turned back to focus on the road. There was a garbage truck in front of him. He changed lanes to get around the truck, but the truck driver crossed in front of him. "Damn, a garbage truck in the third lane!" he said to himself. Suddenly, a large can, which had been hanging on the truck dislodged and bounced onto the highway just in front of Daniel's car. His eyes widened as he felt blood rush to his head. Daniel tried to reduce his speed and swerved to the left to avoid hitting the can. However, the entire left side of his car scraped the dividing barrier in the middle of the highway. Now, with his heart pounding in his chest, he quickly steered the car to the right. Unfortunately he crashed into another car. Daniel's car was pushed toward the center lane and spun around ninety degrees. Another vehicle unable to avoid the accident, crashed into the front of Daniel's car. "How many more cars are going to hit me?" Daniel thought terrifyingly. He tried to turn his steering wheel to the right, but it was locked in place! He was panicked about the fact that he had lost control of his car. Suddenly, he was thrown forward as the result of an impact to the rear of his car! The air bag inflated at once and pushed him backward. Then, he felt that everything came to halt. Luckily, there were no more impacts to his car. He could hear the traffic and the blasting of some car horns. He was in shock. His hands were trembling and his body felt immobile. He remained inside the car trying to regain his composure. The driver of the garbage truck was gone, not knowing what a mess he had created.

Daniel's car had been hit hard in the collision. Surprisingly, all the windows were intact, except for a crack in the rear one. A few seconds later, someone knocked on the window of Daniel's car.

"Are you OK?" a woman asked.

Daniel pushed the air bag aside, looked at the woman and nodded his head, indicating that he was fine.

The woman tried to open Daniel's driver-side door to allow him to get out, but the semi-demolished door was stuck. Another person tried to open his passenger doors, but that too was impossible. Daniel discovered the control panel for the windows was broken and, thereafter, he was not able to open any of them. Daniel was trapped inside his car! He could see a few people. Some were standing around his car. Others were walking around the scene. After a few minutes, he felt some pain in his hands. When he looked down at them, he found that they were burned as a result of the friction between the wheel and the rapidly inflating of the air bag.

Less than half an hour later, the siren of an ambulance could be heard. Two paramedics emerged from the ambulance and began questioning the spectators to determine what had happened. Daniel could see them through the window, but he could not hear what they were saying. One of the men approached Daniel's car and stood in front of the driver's window, "How are you, sir?"

"I am fine, but I think the doors are locked," Daniel answered.

The paramedic tried to open the driver's door, but was unsuccessful. Then, he moved to the other doors, only to discover they were all locked. The man went to the ambulance and returned with a bat.

"Sir, I have to break the window to get you out," the paramedic informed him. Daniel agreed. The man went to the other side of the car and broke the back passenger window with the bat. After he opened the door, he crawled into the car. As he got close to Daniel, he asked, "Are you OK, sir?"

"I'm alive. I think my hands are burned."

Daniel was taken to the hospital. He was found only to have second-degree burns on his hands and was discharged. He called Isaac, his friend, to come and pick him up. Isaac could not believe that Daniel had escaped with his life from a multiple car accident. Unfortunately, still not appreciating life, Daniel asked Isaac to stop at the nearest store so he could buy a pack of cigarettes on the way home. Before that evening ended, he had finished the pack.

A week later, Daniel came to my office for the follow up on his smoking cessation. His face was pale. His voice was filled with anguish. A dressing of gauze covered each of his hands. Something else was also noticeable; he did not have his tie! He had a devastated appearance.

"Daniel," I asked with concern, "I have never seen you like this! Are you OK?"

"No! Things are not good," he answered with a shaky voice. "I saw the angel of death before my eyes last week."

"What happened to you? Why is there a bandage on your hands?"

"A frigging garbage can almost killed several people. Me included!"

"A garbage can?"

"Doc, I was involved in a horrible car accident! A large can fell off a garbage truck. Right in front of me. In the third lane of the highway! I tried to prevent the accident, but, considering what happened, I'm lucky to be alive!"

With great drama, Daniel unfolded the story of his accident and how he had survived it. I had to let him rest for a while before continuing the session. I was extremely happy to discover that physically he was unharmed, but I realized that, mentally, he was frightened.

"In general, how are you doing with everything else?" I asked him as we changed the subject.

Daniel took a deep sigh and said, "Ah, I'm sorry to let you down this time, but I could not help it."

"What do you mean by that?"

"Doc, I still smoke. Even more than before. About two packs a day!" he said with remorse. "Things are not good now. You know, with this accident, I lost myself. I feel irritated. The problem with my prostate does not help at all. My marital life is going down the drain as well."

At times during an office visit, a physician may choose silence to show compassion or use it to reach a goal. So, I became quiet for a few seconds. Daniel looked at me and asked, "Doc, are you OK"?

"Yes, Daniel, I'm all right. But, I'm worried about you. Things definitely haven't gotten any better."

"I cannot sleep well at night. I get anxious. I have butterflies in my stomach all the times! Things are not easy for me. Do you understand?"

"Daniel, I always understood you. However, I have doubts about whether you are heading in the right direction."

"I appreciate your concern. I try hard to do the right thing. However, this problem concerning my prostate does not give me peace. At night, I might wake up and think about it. I might sweat so much that I have to get up and change my clothes. Unfortunately, it is getting worse every day!"

"I see you are anxious."

"Anxious! Anxious is not the word to explain my condition. I'm super anxious!" he explained. Then he continued, "Do you think that it would be better for me to go for another biopsy earlier? Or should I just wait for a few more months as was planned?"

"I don't think you need to have another biopsy sooner. You'd better wait as the urologist recommended. Regarding your emotional problems, it looks like you are having some panic attacks. If you would like, I can prescribe some medication to improve your anxiety and the sleep."

"No, Doc! I don't like to take medications. Let me take care of it by myself."

Daniel and I stayed in touch over the next two months, either by telephone or face-to-face in my office. Every time, he appeared emotionally drained. The sallow complexion of his face did not disappear. Meanwhile, he found a new urologist to take care of him. Four months after my first evaluation, Daniel called me. "Doc, I had another biopsy this morning. Would you let me know about the report as soon as you get it?"

"How did it go?"

"It was easier than the first time."

"Very well, I'll be in touch with you as soon as they send the report."

Two days later, I received the biopsy report. Contrary to the first report, this one was really easier to comprehend. It was exactly what Daniel never wished for, a "total disaster". He had six biopsies, two of which came back as definitive cancer! Thus, I asked him to see me for a follow-up visit.

"Are you sure about what you are saying?" Daniel asked me in my office after I showed him the report.

"I'm sure. The question is how you want to approach it," I said. "The treatment is either surgery, radiation, or do nothing."

"Doc, I'm still young! I'm afraid of the surgery! They may possibly cut the nerves and I might become impotent! I did my own investigation already."

"That's right. There are some risks involved."

"What do you suggest?"

"It is truly up to you. My best recommendation is for you to become familiar with all the options. Then, make a decision. Let's talk about it again after you visit the urologist."

Daniel was bewildered when he left my office. The uncertainty about his diagnosis was ended. Now, he had to make a decision about his future. Becoming impotent for a man of his age was tremendously frightening and could break him emotionally. Furthermore, radiation therapy, such as seed implantation, or receiving hormonal treatment, had other problems. To make it more complicated, he could take no action beyond regular follow-up visits.

Daniel was highly motivated and interested in learning about the different approaches to the treatment of prostate cancer. He started talking to his friends, going on the Internet, reading materials and discussing it with his wife. However, his indecision increased as he learned more. Before Daniel made a final decision, Isaac accompanied Daniel to his new urologist. The office was located in a large cancer center. The doctor, who was in his late 30's, recommended a few options, including the new microscopic nerve preservation prostatectomy. This procedure would reduce the likelihood of becoming impotent, but nothing was guaranteed. Daniel was apprehensive about being operated on by a young physician. However, he had to make a choice and hope for the best.

Against all odds, and despite Daniel's beliefs, one month after his diagnosis, the young urologist operated on him. On the day of the surgery, Daniel's wife, Sandra, and his friend, Isaac, waited impatiently at the hospital for a few hours until he was brought into the recovery room. During the next few hours, analgesics helped him to cope with the pain. He experienced anxiety over the possible loss of his manhood, a very vital psychological element for a man.

Three weeks after the surgery, Daniel came to see me for a benign pain in his ear. He appeared surprisingly well. He was cheerful and his lips were pinkish color. He surprised me with his comments when I asked him questions. "You look much better than during your previous visits. Did you do anything new, besides your recent surgery?" I asked.

"Doc, finally, I did the right thing. It's already been a month since I've smoked my last cigarette!" he answered proudly.

A big smile appeared on my face. "A month!" I said, "That is incredible! You really did need a big impact or a catastrophe to make you stop smoking."

"Well, Doc, I had to do what I had to do. Cigarettes were my friend, but I had enough of it."

"You are giving me good news. I'm also glad that your operation went well, without complications," I commented.

"Me, too!" he said, "You don't know what I went through! Hopefully, it is all over. However, I still sweat at nights, my sleep is disturbed, and my wife is hysterical about everything."

"Wah! Sounds terrible!" I said.

"Believe me, it is hard. But I'm working on It. Let's hope for the best."

After I finished examining him and writing a prescription for his earache, he looked at me and said, "I owe you one. You saved my life! If it weren't for you, I would have never known that I had prostate cancer. Your finger is worth a million!"

◆   ◆   ◆

Daniel ended his tobacco use after a life-altering roller coaster ride and a challenge with prostate cancer. Once, smoking was called a psychologically dependent habit. Later on, after discovering a multitude of chemicals in cigarettes, doctors were led to new ideas concerning the chemical dependency to tobacco. This by itself guided many pharmaceutical companies to manufacture different medications to help patients who wanted to end their habit. However, I believe smoking should be considered a disease as a separate entity, or a subcategory of a larger group of diseases of chemical dependency, like the dependency to drugs and alcohol. Some human beings have weaknesses and needed to comfort themselves by "drugs". In simple terms, it sounds as if there might be "cracks" in the human pleasure-control centers of individuals who are attracted to chemicals. Many companies, such as those in the tobacco industry, gain billions of dollars every year because they are aware of such "cracks". By keeping in mind the concept of a "disease", instead of "dependency", many physicians possibly will have a more effective role in managing smoking cessation. They may do this by empowering the patient with interest to deviate from unwanted chemical dependencies.

As for Daniel, he did well after his operation. He never returned to smoking. His will power finally defeated his unwanted desires and brought him to triumph. Nine months after his surgery, though he came to visit me for a repeated ear infection, our main conversation was about his challenges. Although he was still obese, he looked wonderful, full of energy, and optimistic about his future. He even started a new business. When I asked him about his marital life, he said, "Doc, we are going to a marriage counselor! It costs a fortune, but it is truly worth it! By the way, I'm very lucky. I was always scared about becoming impotent, but it never happened to me. I have more than 90% erection with good sexual satisfaction. Life is much better now." As I listened to him, I enjoyed the successful story of his life and how he accomplished his goals. For my part, I was happy to provide him with an opportunity to have a longer life by discovering his cancer in its early stage. I was also delighted to support him in the various challenges that he had to go through. Hopefully, I will be able to provide him with support for other challenges in the years to come!

MEDICAL WISDOM

Prostate cancer is diagnosed in more than 200,000 American men every year. More than 41,000 individuals may die annually from prostate cancer, making it the second leading cause of cancer death in men after lung cancer. Prostate cancer is more prevalent in black men than in white men and is diagnosed at later stages in black men[5]. A man with two or more affected first-degree relatives has a higher risk of developing this disease. Prostate cancer is more common in advanced age, but is rarely diagnosed in men under age 50. The possibility of developing prostate cancer increases as the age of men advances. This is a slow growing cancer with its expansion being influenced by testosterone (male hormones). The reduction in the level of this hormone, as it might occur in older age or with certain treatments, decreases the progression of the disease in ones who already suffer from prostate cancer.

Prostate cancer does not show any signs or symptoms in early stages. As the disease progresses, the cancer may cause an enlargement of the prostate or spread to different parts of body (metastases), such as bones and lymph nodes. About 60% of patients with prostate cancer have advanced or metastatic disease at the time of diagnosis. Presence of blood in the urine or growing pain in the lower back could represent some of the symptoms in advanced cases.

Early detection of prostate cancer is important in order to prevent a poor outcome in the progressive stages of the disease. Yet, there is no definitive screening test for this type of malignancy. Tests currently used are the *digital rectal exam* (DRE), *prostate specific antigen* (PSA) and *transrectal ultrasound.*

DRE is usually started between the ages of 40–50 and may be performed annually in the physician's office. The sensitivity of this test increases with a more "experienced gloved index finger".

The PSA is a blood test. Its level might be normal in the early stage of prostate cancer, but may rise with pathological processes, such as in advanced malignancy, inflammation, or benign enlargement of the prostate. These characteristics make the PSA not a very sensitive screening test. A rise in the PSA level over time might signify a development of an abnormality in the prostate tissue. Performing regular tests every year or two, in suspicious cases of prostate cancer, may be considered a good means for follow up.

Ultrasound is used in cases where the diagnosis is in doubt. Although inconvenient, this is used mostly to guide prostate biopsies. A positive pathological biopsy report is the definitive method to make a true diagnosis. Infection and bleeding are potential risks of having a biopsy.

Limitations in each of the cancer screening methods may lead to discrepancies in recommendations from different professional review groups. For example, US Preventive Service Task Force does not recommend any routine population-screening test for prostate cancer[23]. On the other hand, the American Cancer Society recommends annual DRE and PSA, beginning at the age of 50, for men who have at least a 10-year life expectancy, and at the age of 45 for high risks patients. Given the lack of a universal recommendation, decisions about screening must be made on an individual basis.

There are three options of treatment for prostate cancer. These are based on the stage of progression of the disease, the patient's age, and his wishes. These options include 1) surgery, 2) radiation therapy (either external beam or internal seed implants), 3) hormone therapy or orchiectomy (excision of testicles). A fourth choice might be some combination of the major procedures. Some urologists feel that, for older men, the risks of surgery or radiation treatment outweigh any benefits. Therefore, they recommend "watchful waiting", which includes monitoring tumor progression and treatment only in cases of advancing disease. At the present time, randomized trials are in progress to evaluate the efficacy of each treatment. Current recommendations for therapy may change with better data from those trials.

The question remains how can prostate cancer be prevented. Men with a strong family history of prostate cancer and those of the black race may need to pay more attention to their prostate. As it was mentioned, age is a risk factor for prostate cancer. Heavy metal exposure, such as cadmium (an element found in some batteries), vasectomy, and multiple sexual partners are presumably other factors, which increase the risk of this malignancy. A balanced diet (low in fat and animal protein, rich in fiber, vitamin A and D, yellow and green vegetables, and fruits) may help reduce the risk of developing prostate cancer. A weaker association has been found between lower socioeconomic status, occupation, cigarette smoking, prostate enlargement, hormonal levels and the onset of this disease.

◆   ◆   ◆

Obesity is a serious health problem. It increases the potential of developing other diseases, such as heart disease, hypertension, diabetes, respiratory diseases, blood clots, stroke, skin diseases, and even death.

Obesity is a disease that must be controlled as early as childhood. Overweight children have greater risk of developing type II diabetes earlier in their lives (see chapter 12). This was previously considered an adult-onset disease[6]. Boys with chubby bellies are also more likely to have high blood pressure than their slimmer counterparts[7].

In adults, elevated blood pressure can be the consequence of being overweight. In addition, obesity may cause sleep apnea, a medical issue, which also may lead to high blood pressure. Elevated blood pressure may lead to heart disease, kidney disease, problems with the vision and many others. The formation of blood clots in the legs and developing a stroke are also linked to obesity. The blood clots in the legs may travel to the lungs, causing a condition called pulmonary embolism, resulting in high blood pressure in the lungs, or even sudden death[6]. Many infections of the skin such, as fungal infections, may develop in skin folds of obese patients. Elderly, bed-ridden, obese patients are at high risk of developing pressure ulcers, a debilitated problem.

Education about following a healthy diet has to begin in early childhood. Parents must be encouraged to avoid so called "junk foods" in their children's diet. Teachers may also play an active role in this teaching process with their students. Physicians, perhaps, should pursue the guidelines of a healthy diet for overweight adults although the weight-lowering process might be slow. Regular exercises, also, have to be included in every obese patient's regimen.

◆   ◆   ◆

Accidents, in general, are the leading cause of death among the young population. **Motor vehicle accidents** are one of the reasons for death and disability among teens. Almost half of all automobile-related teenage deaths involve drunk drivers. Using seat belts is important for protection. Since the seats in a car are secured to the body, they are usually not damaged in a crash. The same rule, therefore, applies for persons who secure themselves with seat belts. As a driver, assure the safety of all passengers by requiring the use of their seat belts. Also, driving a medium or a large sized car may give you an added protective layer.

Although unpredictable, many car accidents are preventable if we know what factors carry the potential of producing them. Driving under the influence of drugs, alcohol, or even tobacco may jeopardize the driver and the passengers. Eating, using a cellular phone, or having an argument while driving, increases the risk of car accidents. Driving in rain or snow should be minimized to lessen the possibility of motor vehicle collisions.

As a personal reminiscence, back in 1996, after a heavy snowfall, I was driving in the third lane of a highway. Suddenly, a large chunk of ice separated from the roof

of another car in the opposite traffic line. The ice crashed into my windshield, caus-
ing a big crack in the window. Luckily, I was able to control the car to avoid any
accidents. Since then, I do not drive in close proximity to those cars with heavy ice
coating on their roofs.

Securing any item, which is carried on the roof of the car, to prevent their accidental fall, is recommended. Obviously, do not secure the snow and ice on the roof of your car, but remove it completely!! Interestingly, some states in this country have certain rules about leaving ice and snow on your car, and you might get a ticket for not cleaning it.

◆   ◆   ◆

Daniel had many mid-life challenges—smoking cessation, lowering his weight,
treating his prostate cancer, and improving his relationship with his wife. He
Indeed overcame most of them as he found his hidden will power. In his case, as in
many other cases, an achievement is the matter of strong desire. If Daniel changed
his direction and enhanced his health condition by eliminating the undesirable
habits, you will be able to do the same.

7

Life is not Over Until It is Over

1991

Ronald Mantel, a 76 years old man, and his wife, Vivian, were spending a few days away from home at a hotel on a mini-vacation. On the second night, Ronald rose quietly from the bed, and in the dark room, made his way to the restroom. He did not turn on the light fearing he might disturb his wife, who was sleeping in bed. In the restroom, the dim light was enough for him to see around. When he started passing his urine, he experienced some unusual feeling. When he finished, he switched on the light. He looked in the bowel and saw that the water was bloody. "I probably passed something," he thought to himself. He shrugged his shoulders, flushed the lavatory, and returned to his bed.

Ronald did not seek any medical attention concerning his bloody urine until it happened again six months later. Then, he thought, "Probably something is going on!" After he saw a urologist he discovered that he was suffering from prostate cancer.

"What do you want to do, Ronald?" the urologist asked when Ronald visited him in his office.

"I don't know! You are the doctor! You have to tell me!" Ronald said.

"Well, the best treatment that I suggest for you is orchiectomy."

"What is that?"

"This means removal of your testicles!"

"Ooh, this is painful. Why do you have to do that?"

"Your male hormone is like a food for your garden. With no food, your garden might not bloom, or bloom but just a little bit."

"I understand. I have a garden, full of zucchini and lettuce. I give them water and food all the time. It is the best garden in the neighborhood."

The doctor looked at Ronald's hearing aids and said, "I don't think you understand me. Let me rephrase my sentence…"

Ronald cut him short and said, "Doc, I got you! You said that my male hormone makes the cancer grow. So, by removing my testicles, you get rid of my hormones."

"Walla! You learn fast!" the doctor said, with a smile on his face.

"Doc, you smile!" Ronald said seriously. "But I have to explain to my wife that next month I'll be walking without my testicles!"

"I apologize. I really didn't mean to hurt your feelings!"

Ronald laughed sarcastically. "I am joking with you, Doc! It has already been a couple of years since my sex life became non-existent! I fully understand you. Whatever you say, Doc. So, when do you want to cut me?"

"You not only learn fast, you like to act fast!"

1996

In the winter of 1996, I joined the practice of an elderly physician. He had to take a long leave of absence due to an illness. It was a good opportunity for me to practice medicine in a different perspective. It was during that time that I met Ronald's wife, Vivian. Her personal assistant, Margaret, a woman in her 50's, accompanied Vivian to the appointment. As I entered the exam room, I saw Vivian sitting on the examination table. She was an old, frail lady. Her back and neck were bent, her teeth appeared to be loose, and her eyes were covered with large thick glasses.

"Doctor T, Vivian doesn't feel well," Margaret said passionately. "She is not steady on her feet and leans toward the right when she stands."

"How long has she been like this?" I asked.

"For a while…a day or two!" Margaret answered.

As I studied Vivian's chart, I discovered that she had multiple diseases, including high blood pressure and heart disease. She required numerous medications. Since she lacked specific symptoms and I had a great deal of difficulty comprehending the hand written notes of her former physician, I was compelled to ask Margaret and Vivian a series of questions.

"How do you feel, ma'am?" I asked Vivian.

"Ooh, I'm dizzy. Just like this, look…" she said, and let herself lean to the right. She would have fallen to the floor if Margaret and I had not grabbed hold of her.

Once we stabilized Vivian on the examination table, I asked Margaret, "Does she take her medications regularly?"

"Oh, doctor, of course. I give them to her every day," she replied with pride.

"How is her appetite?" I asked.

"Terrible. Terrible, doctor! She just doesn't want to eat or drink," Margaret said with concern.

"I'm just not hungry," Vivian interrupted.

I asked many other questions in order to determine the main problem. It was during my examination that I discovered Vivian's blood pressure was very low. This is a condition which can occur easily in elderly people who lack sufficient fluid intake. I informed Margaret that I would adjust some of her medications to improve her low blood pressure and I encouraged her to drink fluids. Some blood tests, as well as other diagnostic tests, such as computerized tomography of her head were necessary for a full evaluation. I scheduled her for a follow-up appointment as well.

The extent of the work-up and the care I showed impressed Ronald. Several days passed before I had an opportunity to speak with Ronald.

"I'm calling to inform you about the report of the CT of Vivian's head," I said. "Everything is good. It showed that she had a stroke in the past. This does not have anything to do with her current condition."

"Thank you for your call, doctor. I think you did a good job. She is doing much better since you changed her medications. She tries to eat better, too."

"Well, if there are any other problems, please let me know."

"OK! I'll do that. Thank you again, and God bless you."

When Vivian came back for her follow-up, she still appeared very weak. She remained unsteady on her feet and needed Margaret and Ronald to help her walk. Surprisingly, she was completely alert.

"Hello, Mrs. Mantel," I said as I entered the exam room.

"Oh, hello! Hello! You look nice! I like your outfit," she said with a smile.

"Thank you for your compliment. How do you feel today?"

"Oh, you know! I'm the same old lady."

"Doctor T. She's really doing better. But, you know, she recently has become forgetful," Ronald said.

"Problems don't stop! How is her dizziness?" I asked.

"To be honest with you, she has gotten dizzy on and off for the past few months. But, this time it was worse," Ronald said.

The facts were slowly falling into place. I was beginning to visualize a better picture of what was happening to Vivian. Her symptoms had existed for a long time, probably for months. This fact made it clear that she was an elderly woman experiencing gradual deterioration. I felt obligated to help her and Ronald go through a very difficult period. However, even with my best intentions, my work would terminate unfinished, since I had to leave that practice when the other physician resumed his work schedule.

1997

One cold winter day, I received a call at home from Ronald.

"Dr. T. This is Mr. Mantel. Do you remember me?"

"Mr. Mantel! Hi! How are you? It has been a long time since I've heard from you. Of course, I remember you! How is your wife?"

"Oh, I'm so glad that I could find you. About my wife! This is exactly what I wanted to discuss with you. Her legs are swollen. I'd like to ask you to come and visit her at our house. Is that possible for you?"

"I thought that she sees her primary physician for her medical problems!"

"No, forget about him. He doesn't do any more house calls. That's why I'm asking you to come."

"Ronald, as you know, I do not have my own practice in this area."

"That's OK. I don't mind. However, because we know you, and you know us, I thought that you might be the best person to help us."

Finally, as a result of Ronald's persistence, I agreed to see Vivian at home. Ronald tried to give me the direction to his house. "You will see an American flag on a tall pole in my front yard. No one else in the neighborhood has this," he explained proudly over the phone.

I drove to the Mantels' residence. I recognized their house easily as I pulled up the driveway. When I came close to the entrance door, a dog began barking. Ronald opened the door very gently as he tried to halter his large brownish dog. As I entered the small living room, I saw Vivian. She was seated on a comfortable looking sofa next to the fireplace. She was wrapped with a blue blanket around her shoulders. She appeared happy to see me. Margaret was also there. She was definitely a wonderful help to Vivian and an emotional support for Ronald. She rose from her chair to welcome me.

A house call for a physician can be a very exciting visit to evaluate a patient in his or her natural surroundings. This environment usually contains many elements that cannot be identified during an office visit. In the case of Vivian, I learned that the scale of her mobility was limited because of the small size of her house.

As I examined Vivian, I noticed that not only her legs were swollen, but also she had some difficulty breathing. I discovered that her symptoms were related to congestive heart failure, a condition in which the heart cannot adequately force the blood out. I reviewed her medications and recognized that I had to adjust her water pills. As I sat down next to the table to write a few prescriptions, Ronald left the house. When he returned, he had several wood sticks in his hands. As he threw them into the fireplace, I made a comment, "You need to have plenty of sticks to keep the fire going!"

"Oh, I have as much as I want. I have enough for at least 3 more years," Ronald said.

"It is good to be warm," Vivian said with a smile.

As I was finishing my house call, I encouraged Margaret to help Vivian walk as much as possible. I handed the prescriptions to Ronald and explained the directions about taking the medications. Ronald expressed his appreciation for my visit. As I opened the door to leave, the cold wind brushed my face. It was then that I realized how warm it was inside the house.

A few days later, when I spoke to Ronald, it was nice to hear that Vivian's swelling of her legs had improved.

I was enjoying a relaxing Sunday morning. A heavy snow had covered the ground from the night before. It was less than a month since I visited Vivian. The house phone rang. It was Margaret.

"Dr. T, Vivian can't breathe well! She just doesn't look right!" she said.

"Are you giving her the medications as I directed?"

"Yes, of course. Her legs got swollen again and her appetite is not great. Would you come to see her in the house again?" she asked nicely.

"Apparently, she needs another visit. OK, I'll come, but it might take a while before I get there because of the heavy snow."

"That's fine, as long as you can get here, it would be fine," Margaret said with a sigh of relief.

This time locating Vivian's house was not as easy as the first time due to the snow covering everything. It took me a long time because I drove slowly. This was a good opportunity for me to think what other venues were left for me to ease her problems. As I parked my car next to her house, Margaret opened the door. It appeared she had been waiting for me. As I expected, the dog came to the door, too, but this time he did not bark even once. He went to the corner of the room and sat down. Vivian was in her usual spot, next to the fireplace.

"Hello, Dr. T. It is nice to see you here," Vivian said.

"Hello, Vivian. Where is Ronald?" I asked.

"Oh, he went to bring in some logs from outside," Margaret explained.

"So, how is my lady doing?" I asked.

"I'm OK. I feel good," Vivian said as she scratched her back.

"It is good to hear that," I said as I studied Vivian. She did not seem to be in any distress, but both legs appeared to be swollen as I glanced at them. Before I finished my thoughts, Ronald entered, holding a bunch of kindling.

"Dr. T, you are here! I'm so glad to see you," he said.

"Thank you, Ronald. How are you?"

"Oh, I'm good. I'm always good," he said as he put the sticks into the fireplace. "You know Dr. T, I'm 80 years old and I have never been worried. That's why I'm always good! Even when I was diagnosed with prostate cancer I was not worried."

"That's a great outlook," I said. "Well, let's take care of the lady."

"Have you opened your own practice already?" he asked me.

"Oh, not yet. We are in its building process." I explained. "Hopefully, soon, my office will be open."

"That's great. I'm sure you are going to be successful," Ronald said.

"Thank you," I said.

As I finished examining Vivian, I did not find any overt difficulty in breathing, but she did have many scratch marks on her back and arms. I sat at the table to review her chart, which I carried with me. Ronald sat in front of me on the other side. As I was looking at the list of her medications to refresh my mind, Ronald said, "Dr. T, you have to help her. She itches like crazy."

"Yah, I see that. How long has she been scratching herself?" I asked.

"Oh, quite a while. Isn't that right, Margaret?" he said as he looked at Margaret.

"Yes, it's already a few weeks. We are using the hydrocortisone cream all the time, but it doesn't work. Do you have any better idea for her?" Margaret asked.

"She had the same problem a few years ago. So, we took her to the dermatologist. He diagnosed her with eczema. He prescribed this cream," said Ronald as he handed me a tube of potent steroid cream.

Family members who care for a sick person at home may feel desperate as unusual symptoms appear during the course of an illness. They desperately seek a solution to make their loved one comfortable. This was happening to the Mantels. I understood that the itching was the main reason for requesting me to visit Vivian rather than her shortness of breath. I was wondering what I could do for her beyond the treatment with the hydrocortisone cream that she was already receiving. The appearance of her skin made me speculate about a different condition beyond a simple eczema.

"Ronald, Vivian probably needs to be evaluated. With this cream, if she doesn't get any better, you must take her to a dermatologist," I said.

"Where do we have to take her?" he asked.

"Maybe to the same dermatologist who saw her before?"

"So, you don't prescribe any cream to relive her symptoms! You know, doctor, it is very difficult to take her out of the house in this weather. Can't you just prescribe another cream to relieve her symptoms?" he asked.

"I understand, but her problem might be beyond a simple eczema," I said. "With all the medications that she is on, she needs a blood test, too."

"OK, doctor," he said. "I'll take her to the dermatologist."

Four days later, I received a telephone page from Dr. Greenberg, the dermatologist who saw Vivian.

"Dr. T, I saw your patient, Mrs. Mantel, in my office 4 days ago. The visit concerned her itching. I took the liberty of performing a blood test on her. You know, her BUN and creatinine were high," he said. Then, he read the numbers to explain that her kidney function had deteriorated tremendously because of lack of fluids.

"Oh, this is not good. You know she suffers from heart failure and she is on diuretics. She needs to pass more urine, otherwise she gets shortness of breath," I said.

"Yeah, that's right," he said.

"So, her itching is the systemic presentation of her kidney failure," I said.

"It appears so," he said. "Any more of the diuretics may aggravate the condition of her kidneys. Unfortunately, as you said, she needs those medications because of her heart condition."

"That puts her in a very difficult position," I said. "On one hand, the medications made her dry, but on the other hand, without those medications, she developed shortness of breath and an increase in the swelling of her legs."

"I don't know what else to do, except suggesting adjustment of her treatment and using a soothing cream," he said.

"Well, I'll try to work on it," I said.

After I hung up the phone, I was happy that I had a clue about Vivian's problem. However, it made me sad to know that Vivian was suffering from kidney failure. I thought about her condition, "She already had a stroke, her heart was weak, and her kidneys were in a bad shape. What else is left? Damn! These water pills! They can be good, but at the same time they may cause harm!" Then, suddenly, something clicked in my mind. The fireplace! I remembered the long hours Vivian spent next to the fireplace without moving. She sat there all day long during the wintertime. "The water pills made her dry, but the heat coming out of the fire place made her even more dry!" I thought with anguish.

Vivian, without knowing about any of the new information, still enjoyed her quality hours next to the fireplace. She continued to do so even after I disclosed the information regarding her kidneys to Ronald. Nothing was changed except that I modified her medication to prevent any further decline in her health condition. I continued my monthly visits to the Mantel's house to evaluate Vivian and keep her in the best possible shape. However, Vivian, an old lady with minimal reserve continued to deteriorate.

Three months later, Ronald called on the phone to notify me that one of the Vivian's legs was more swollen than the other. I realized that this was not the "usual" swelling of her legs, but something new had developed. "Mr. Mantel, take her to the hospital," I said on the phone.

"To the hospital? Do you think it is so serious?"

"With so many hours of sitting and not moving much, and swelling of one leg only, I suspect she might have a blood clot in her leg."

"Oh, that's what you mean. OK, doctor, I'll take her right away."

When I examined Vivian in the hospital I found her to be very weak. I also noticed that she was suffering from shortness of breath, which appeared unusual to me. I was afraid a blood clot might have traveled to her lungs, too. This is a condition called pulmonary embolism. I ordered a few tests after my visit so that I could support my speculations. As a loyal husband whose main concern was always the safety of his wife, Ronald remained in the hospital. Around 6:30 p.m., Vivian was taken to the radiology department to be tested.

A few minutes before 8:00 p.m., I received a call from the hospital. A Russian-accented medical intern was informing me regarding Vivian's condition and the results of the tests.

"Dr. Tabib, this is Mary Kapolsky. I'm the medical intern taking care of Mrs. Mantel."

"Hi, Mary. Do you have any new information about Mrs. Mantel?"

"As a matter of fact, yes. She has DVT[1] in the right leg and numerous pulmonary emboli scattered in both lungs," she said. Her voice was filled with concern about the safety of Vivian's life because of the location of these blood clots.

"Oh, that's what I was afraid of. How is she doing now?"

"She looks OK. But we are afraid she might throw more emboli to the lungs."

---

1.   DVT—deep vein thrombosis is formation of blood clot in the deep venous system.

"You are definitely right! She probably needs an IVC^2 filter to prevent more embolism migration."

"I think you are right."

"Does the husband agree with the procedure?"

"I don't know. I haven't spoken to him about this yet. Actually, he is sitting in a chair next to the patient. Do you want me to call him, so you can discuss the matter with him?"

"That would be great. Let me talk to him."

It did not take long before Ronald got on the phone with me.

"Hi, Ronald. This is Dr. Tabib."

"Dr. T, it's good to hear you. How are you?" he asked.

"I'm fine. I'm concerned about your wife," I said passionately.

"Oh, she is a sick lady. What do you think it is?"

"Ronald, she has a blood clot in the leg and several more blood clots in the lungs. We can give her medications to make her blood thin or insert a filter into the vein that carries blood to the heart to prevent migration of the blood clots. Or, we could do both. Each one of these methods has some advantages and disadvantages. With blood thinners, there is a risk of bleeding. The insertion of a filter is a surgical procedure with its own risks. I wanted you to be informed about these treatments. Do you have any preference regarding these procedures?"

"I don't know. I'm not a doctor! You are!"

"Do you mean that you want me to make a decision about your wife?"

"You know better. That's why I chose you as our doctor. To make decisions! I go along with whatever you say, Doc," he answered firmly.

Since Ronald was unable to choose between the proposed types of medical care, I was put in an awkward position. I was accustomed to the system that allows the patients or their family members to select the type of medical care. In this case, I was asked to make a decision! As I was holding the phone receiver, I thought, "What kind of treatment would I choose if Vivian was my mother?" Even with such a question, no definitive answer came to my mind. Now, it was obvious to me that it was much easier to ask the family member to make a decision rather than to put the burden on the physician. As Vivian's physician, I had the responsibility of being in charge of her life, a duty that I had carried with me concerning every patient of mine. The difference was, in this case, the burden of the responsibility seemed heavier.

---

2.   IVC—inferior vena cava. This is a large vein, which brings the blood from the lower part of the body back to the heart.

"OK, Ronald. I feel that the best choice is to put a filter in the vein. This way, we hopefully can prevent any further problem," I said.

"Doc, I agree with whatever you choose," Ronald said.

"OK, so let me talk to the intern to proceed with the plan," I said.

When I spoke to the intern, I told her about my arrangement with Ronald. In response, she agreed to call the radiologist for insertion of the filter that same night. As Ronald told Vivian about what we decided to do, she just said, "OK, whatever!" It was just before 9:00 p.m. when Vivian was taken to the radiology department for the procedure. Ronald, who had a full commitment to his wife, stayed behind closed doors until she was brought out from the surgical room. "She is OK," the radiologist said when he saw Ronald waiting outside. Around 10:00 p.m., the same intern called me to let me know about the successful outcome of the procedure.

The next day I went to see Vivian in the hospital. Margaret and Ronald were at her bedside. They both smiled as I entered the room. Vivian appeared thin and fragile. On the bed, she was lying on her side in a fetal position with her legs bent toward her abdomen.

"Hello, Dr. T. How are you doing?" said Ronald with a big smile on his face.

"Hello, Mr. Mantel. Hello, Margaret," I responded.

"She is doing much better, thank God," said Margaret happily.

Then, a weak but excited voice came from Vivian, "Hi, Dr. T."

I got closer to the bed and looked at Vivian. I held her hand gently and I asked, "Hello, Vivian. How is my lady?"

She slightly turned her eyes toward me, and without moving any other parts of her body, said in a tiny voice, "I'm fine."

As I was finishing up my visit, Ronald asked, "Dr. T, when do you think we can take her home?"

"As soon as possible."

"I think we need a hospital bed in the house. She is weak," Margaret said passionately. "She cannot move much any more,"

"I agree with you. I'll speak to the care manager to arrange this."

"Thank you Dr. T."

As I left the room, a wave of sadness came over my body. To see the worsening of a patient of mine was always difficult for me. In the last two years, I had seen Vivian deteriorate. By being bed ridden, I realized that her possibilities of revitalization had declined tremendously. With all the rewards and support that a physician may receive from the family members, especially during the difficult periods of treating a patient, geriatric medicine has a painful touch at times.

I visited Vivian in her house two weeks after her discharge from the hospital. It was not surprising to me that she had developed bedsores in her buttocks. "Dr. T, it is all red," said Margaret, with despair, as she pulled down Vivian's diaper.

"Yes, indeed, it is red! It looks like she has some yeast infection, too," I said sadly.

Ronald, who stood next to us, shook his head and then said with a sigh, "Ah, there is no end to it."

After we left the room, I sat with Ronald at the table to discuss the treatment. He shocked me with his question, "Dr. T, do you think she can make it?"

I knew Ronald as a man who could jest at times, but now, there was no joke. "Are you worried?" I asked with concern.

"You know me. I'm never worried. But, I look at her and I see that she is failing. I just want to know if I'm right."

"I think you are right. Is there anything that you want to do?"

"She never wanted to be in this shape," he said softly, with a profound sadness. "She always told me to keep her comfortable. As you know, we never had any children. So, we relied on each other all our lives. We promised each other not to let either one of us suffer when the time comes. Now, I think the time has come!"

I heard the words "promise", "suffering", and "to keep her comfortable". They began whirling around inside my head. The pen I held between my fingers slipped onto the table. I leaned back in the chair and looked down for a few seconds. I could not say a word. For me, Ronald appeared to be a sensible and practical man. I understood that the subject of the discussion was not only about the end of Vivian's life, but also about the end of her *"quality of life."* I looked at Ronald deeply and thought about how lonely he would be without Vivian.

"So, what do you plan to do?" I asked Ronald.

"I don't think I'd hospitalize her any more," he answered. "It will be very tough on her, always sticking her with needles, moving her around from floor to floor and doing procedures. I think enough is enough! Now, she has to be comfortable."

"It looks like you have come to realize that nature has to take its course." A deep sigh ended my sentence.

"Oh, yes," he nodded. "The man has to keep his promises, so do I. I told her a long time ago that I would keep her at ease as she asked me. And, I intend to do so!"

"So, from now on, do you agree with me to try to deliver the treatment for comfort care to her?"

"That's fair enough."

During the next two months, with each visit, I was witness to Vivian's deterioration. Despite the addition of nutritional supplements, she became thinner and thinner. Ronald stayed at her bedside, day and night, as the most faithful husband. He fed her at times, but Vivian's food intake became less and less every day. Whenever he felt that her mouth looked dry, he made it moist with a swab. Many times he sat down next to her bed and recalled various memories that he had shared with her through more than fifty years of a wonderful marriage. However, Vivian was vanishing before his eyes, like a burning candle.

It was a rainy night when Ronald called his nephew, Paul. He lived a few blocks away. Ronald asked him to come to his house.

"Uncle Ron, is every thing OK?" Paul asked.

"Would you come here tonight? I don't feel comfortable."

"What's happening?"

"I don't know. She has a slight fever and she doesn't breathe well."

"Let's see. It's almost 10:00 o'clock," Paul said and looked outside through the window. "Wow! What a rain! OK, uncle, let me finish up with my kids. I'll get there as soon as possible."

"Thank you, Paul."

Less than half an hour later Paul arrived at his uncle's house. As Paul entered the house, Ronald said, "Come in. Look at you! You are all wet! I'm so sorry to put you through so much trouble."

"That's OK. I'm sure that you had good reasons for asking me to be with you tonight. How is she doing?" he asked.

Ronald shook his head and said sadly, "Not good. Not good at all."

Paul took off his raincoat and then walked through a small hallway to get to Vivian's room. "Oh, she doesn't look good! I see that you put the oxygen mask on her, too," Paul said.

"Yeah, I felt she needed that. As a paramedic, you have seen these cases before, haven't you?"

"You are right. I've seen it already. Did she eat today?"

"Yes, but she won't take anything more. She doesn't even accept the moist swabs."

"OK. I think it is best to make the light dim to let her rest. What do you say, uncle?"

"I think you are right."

"Do you want to stay here?" Paul asked passionately, while he gently laid his hand on Ronald's back.

"Yes. I'm comfortable. I wish she would be comfortable, too."

"Take it easy, uncle. You know, maybe I should go and make some coffee for both of us."

Ronald kept studying Vivian's face and then replied, "OK."

As Ronald sat down next to Vivian's bed, he caressed her hands gently. Then, he rose from the chair and looked at her again. He nodded his head and took a deep breath. Finally, he left the room to join Paul in the kitchen.

"For the last few months, she just lies down in the bed. This is not life," Ronald said bitterly as he entered the kitchen.

"Uncle, I think you did the best for her. That's how life is at the end!" Paul said as he put down the cup on the counter.

"It is just not fair to her!" Ronald said, with a quiver in his voice.

The hands of the clock were getting close to midnight. The sound of a heavy downpour and the rustle of the wind filled the house. Ronald paced impatiently in the hallway. He turned and walked into Vivian's room. He stood at the end of her bed and studied her. Suddenly, a flash of lightning penetrated through the window and revealed her drawn, thin face. Ronald raised both his hands and said loudly, "Go, Vivian! Go, Vivian! Please, go now!" Suddenly, an echo of thunder rumbled in the air. Ronald brought his hands down. He took a step backward, and, as sorrow gripped him, his teardrops fell to the floor. A few minutes later, with her last breath, Vivian's soul peacefully left her body.

◆   ◆   ◆

The next day, when I heard the news of Vivian's passing, I went to see Ronald at his home. Margaret, who was cleaning the house, greeted me. "Where is Ronald?" I asked.

"He has gone to take care of the funeral?"

"How is he doing?"

"Oh, he is handling it very well."

"Were you here last night?"

"No, I was in my house. But, I heard that he had a rough time last night. It was ironic with the rain. Even the sky was crying."

I sat with Margaret for a while to comfort her. We discussed Vivian's life in the recent years.

Later that afternoon, Ronald called me.

"Dr. T, I heard that you came by this morning to see me. I'm sorry that I missed you," he said.

"Me, too! How are you doing?" I asked.

"I'm fine. Unfortunately, she is gone. But, I'm glad that she is resting in peace now," he said.

"I'm sure that she will be missed."

"She was a good wife. We had a good time together. But, life goes on!"

"I'm glad to hear optimism in your voice."

"Oh, always! Listen, I want to express my appreciation for all your help in the last two years. You helped my wife and me to go through a rough time. I thank you. Especially for the numerous house calls that you made. I'll never forget your kindness."

"Oh, you're welcome. I wish I could have done more."

"God bless you!"

"We will be in touch."

"Definitely!" he said softly.

Ronald had never left Vivian's bedside when she was ill. With Vivian's death, Ronald's life headed to a different direction. He had accomplished his promised mission for the end of her life. Now, he was able to take a deep sigh of relief. However, after her death, it was amazing to see how he overcame his grief during the next few months. Ronald became one of the favorite patrons in my newly opened practice. The bond between us was something beyond the traditional physician-patient relationship. When I saw him in my office for a routine visit about six months after Vivian's death, I asked, "I haven't seen you for a while. Where have you been?"

"I was in Florida to visit my niece," he said cheerfully.

"I see that you are traveling."

"Well, Dr. T, life goes on!" he said with confidence.

"Any new plans?"

"Of course! My next trip is to Alaska."

"Wow! I see someone is having fun!" I said, and he responded with a playful broad smile.

Contrary to my original impression that Ronald would be a lonely man after the death of his wife, he started a new living path. As a matter of fact, he experienced a feeling of fulfillment in accomplishing his commitment to his late wife, not only during her last few years of life, but also through their entire marriage. Ronald continued to travel. Atlantic City, Florida, Upstate New York, and several western states were just a few of the places he visited. He always had a gleeful smile on his face whenever he came back to see me between his trips. In the summer time, he always brought me a few big bunches of zucchini and lettuce from his garden. During every visit he would spread open his arms and repeat his memorable sentence, "I'm OK. I'm never worried. Have you ever seen another person like me? I'm different!"

1999

One day, Margaret called the office to arrange an appointment for Ronald. He was now 84 years old. "What happened to Ronald?" I asked with curiosity.

"He fell on his driveway yesterday and broke his arm," she said.

"Oh! This is terrible. Bring him over now!"

"Don't panic Dr. T. Ronald was already seen by an orthopedist." She tried to calm me, but I was worried for the old man. I asked Margaret to bring him to my office that same day. When I saw him for the evaluation, I noticed a cast. The rest of his arm was all bruised.

"It was a stupid accident! I was just getting out of my car! The next moment I was down on the ground! I don't know how it happened! I assume that I tripped over something as I was getting out of my car," Ronald said.

"Well, you'd better be careful next time when you get out of the car," I said.

"You are right. I have to be more careful," he said. Then, he stretched out his healthy arm and said, "I'm OK. There is no need to worry!"

"I hope you are right. By the way, do you take any calcium supplements?"

"No, I don't take any medicine."

"I advise you to take three calcium pills with vitamin D every day. Eat lots of dairy products to protect your bones."

"I'll do that," he answered.

Then, I wrote in my chart note, "Risk of osteoporosis! Administration of calcium and vitamin D was recommended," and I thought, "Is he really going to be safe?"

When Ronald came back for his follow-up the next month, his fracture was healing. However, he started having stiffness in the shoulder, a problem for which he needed physical therapy. Upon examination, I also noticed his blood pressure was high. I was wondering if he had hypertension, a disease of elevated blood pressure. I scheduled him for another follow up visit and blood tests. When he came back, I had to initiate treatment for his elevated blood pressure. Once I reviewed the test results, I discovered Ronald's prostate cancer had progressed. It looked like he was falling apart, first the fracture of the arm, then hypertension, and now the return of his prostate cancer.

I disclosed the results of the blood tests to Ronald on the phone. Later that day, I received a call from his nephew, Paul.

"Dr. T, I understand that my uncle, Mr. Mantel, has an elevated PSA. Is that correct?" he asked.

"That's correct."

"What do you think we should do?"

"He already has removed his testicles. You'd better take him to the urologist who operated on him to find out if there is anything else left to do for him."

Ronald's visit to the urologist ended up with a new treatment for him. By taking a pill, Ronald would reduce all the remnants of the male hormone that was left in his body. Ronald became very happy when I notified him about the drop in his PSA after six months of that treatment. However, the correction of the numbers did not necessarily mean an improvement in all aspects of his situation. What happened next changed my course of action.

<u>2001</u>

Two years after his first fall, Ronald fell again in the street. A neighbor arranged for him to obtain medical care from his orthopedist. He was in pain when I saw him in the office a few days after the accident. It was heart breaking for me to see Ronald return to my office with a few fractures to his ribs. He assured me that he took his calcium supplements religiously. Apparently, simply taking calcium was not enough to prevent him from experiencing a third fracture of his other arm a few months later. This time he tripped over some object on the lawn next to his house.

Osteoporosis is not an "over night" disease. It develops over the years. During the time I was dealing with Ronald, I attended several seminars about osteoporosis. It became a subject of great interest to me. Osteoporosis is a disease in which bones become weak and fragile. However, most of the information that I gathered concerning this disease was focused on women, but very little on men.

It was at the end of a teaching lecture about osteoporosis that I approached the speaker to inquire about the treatment of this condition in men. He raised his eyebrows and said, "Well, it is not a common practice at this time, but there is a potential to use medications for a subgroup of men." Obviously, Ronald was in my mind!

Even with his advanced age, Ronald was a man full of energy and enthusiasm. He was still eager to travel and enjoy his life. So, I felt that I had the duty to do everything in my power to keep him as healthy as possible, even though I knew he was suffering from the devastating disease of prostate cancer.

At the first opportunity, I suggested to Ronald to have a bone density scan to evaluate the condition of his bones. He welcomed my decision. As soon as I received the report, I called him to come in for a follow-up.

"Hello, Dr. T. How are you doing? How is the family?" he asked.

"Hi, Ron. I'm fine. The family is good, too. How are you?"

Oh, you know me," he said with a big smile, and then spread his arms in his famous gesture and continued, "I'm always good!"

"Well, I have some news for you."

"News! Am I alive?" he asked sarcastically.

"Yes, of course! You are very much alive!"

"Well, tell me. What did you find with my bone density scan?"

"You have been diagnosed with severe osteopenia."

"What is that?"

"This is the step right before you get osteoporosis. It is a decrease in the bone mass."

"Aha!" he answered and looked at me without any emotion. I was wondering if he understood me at all. So I asked, "Have I been clear?"

"Dr. T, I'm listening. I always listen. My hearing aids are working well. I think, you are telling me that my bones are getting weak and that's why they break easily."

"That's quite right," I said.

"Too much medical terminologies!" he said with a laugh. Then he asked, "Any suggestion to correct the problem?"

"Well, there is a relatively new medication on the market that you can take. Its use is actually quite easy. You just have to take it once a week with one full glass of water one hour before breakfast."

"That's easy. Any side effects?"

"It may cause irritation in the lower part of your esophagus, right before the entrance to your stomach,"

Then I pointed to the anatomical chart that was hanging on the wall in my exam room, and showed him the internal organs. I continued, "However, if you take it as I told you the risk of the side effects would be low."

"Dr. T, whatever you say. You are the boss!" he responded.

<u>2002</u>

After Ronald visited his nephew in Florida, he came back to visit me for a blood pressure follow-up. As he entered the exam room, he grasped my hand for a handshake and smiled.

"Hello, Dr. T. I see you have a company. Who is this gentleman?" he asked as he pointed to the person standing next to me.

"This is a medical student who is doing an office rotation with me," I answered, as I introduced the medical student.

"Very nice. I'm glad that you progressed to a point to be able to teach medical students."

Ronald and I chatted about and how enjoyable was his trip. When we finished, he turned to the medical student and said, "He is a great doctor! He helped my wife a lot. I hope that you learn a lot from him."

As Ronald left my office, I thought to myself, which one of us should be more grateful? Me, as a doctor, or Ronald, as a graceful man at his age! He had gone through a very rough time with his wife and, then, emerged proudly! He was living his life very happily with no children and without the presence of his wife at his side. Unknowingly, he taught me a very good lesson. The joy and fulfillment varies in different stages of life. Above all, life is not over until it is over!

MEDICAL WISDOM

Due to advanced technology in this new era of medicine, physicians are able to keep the terminally ill patients alive per their guardian's requests, despite the fact that Mother Nature has been calling them for a long time. Death is an inevitable final point of life. We struggle to postpone the end. The **end-of-life issues** are mostly about the quality of life rather than the quantity. A patient of mine, who was suffering from cancer, said to me, "I don't want to go through chemotherapy. Just imagine, when I die, I won't have to pay taxes! I won't have to shovel the snow in my driveway in winter! I won't have to go grocery shopping or do any more laundry every day! What is better than this?" She actually was saying, "I will be comfortable." This feeling of "comfort" is the issue that a human being has to experience through his or her entire life, especially before death.

Most people in the United States die in the hospital rather than at home or in a nursing home. The hospitalization of terminally ill patients, besides being a huge financial burden on the economy of the country, causes an extreme amount of anxiety for the family members. During the dying process, care has to be extended equally to the patient and the family members. Family members of very sick patients who have multiple medical problems may feel guilty if they do not see their loved ones kept alive mechanically. A physician may offer an essential support to family members by helping them to comprehend that dying is a natural process. Once this step is accomplished, there is often a huge reduction of the remorse felt on behalf of the family. This also eases the physician's task of delivering the appropriate treatment, called **comfort care**. The purpose of this kind of care is to provide the individual with a peaceful death. In this setting, a physician may use morphine or other similar agents to alleviate any possible pain or discomfort the patient may experience in the last days or hours of his or her life. Prolonging of the dying process may cause continuation of suffering for the terminally ill patient and escalation of the anxiety for the family members.

Early on, before the dying process commences, ill patients may reduce the burden of decision making for the next of kin or the guardian by expressing their end of life wishes, either orally or in writing. Legal documents, such as a written advanced directive signed by the patient and two witnesses, or a living will co-signed by an attorney, may instruct a physician about handling the comfort care. In the author's opinion, the choice of how to ease the suffering of a terminally ill patient is a personal issue between the physician, the patient, and the family members. Since there exists a fine line between medical and political issues regarding physician-assisted death and comfort care, those legal documents should clearly define the borders of the treatment rendered to the patient.

A physician has to use his or her medical judgment for elderly ill patients, as well. I recall one occasion when several family members of a patient with a severe systemic infection approached me requesting to end her life by using morphine. I suggested that they withdraw such a decision since I did not feel that was the right time. Sure enough, a year later, I saw the same patient sitting in a wheel chair enjoying the springtime sun in front of a nursing home.

Due to the fact that most terminally ill patients die in a hospital setting, the physician in charge of the case or the family members may receive consultation from the hospital ethics committee if any unanswered questions remain regarding the future of the terminally ill patient. Court orders for the fate of such patients are the last resort.

◆   ◆   ◆

Congestive heart failure means that the heart is unable to pump blood adequately through the body. This leads in congestion, or fluid retention in different parts of the body, such as lungs or legs. As a result of this accumulation of fluids, patients may experience shortness of breath, or heaviness in the legs. Medical treatment is available to alleviate those symptoms. However, many of those patients may require frequent hospitalizations. Living with heart failure can be burdensome for the patient and the family. In mild to moderate cases, patients may suffer from shortness of breath only upon walking, climbing stairs, or during light exercises. As the condition advances, patients may become bed-ridden.

One medication or a combination of medications may be used for the treatment based upon the stage of the heart failure and the patient's other comorbid medical conditions. These medications may have side effects that can be detected by blood tests or by an electrocardiogram. *Diuretics*, frequently called water pills, reduce the accumulation of fluids by increasing urination. *Angiotensin converting enzyme inhibitors* or ACE-I, improve the function of the kidneys by keeping their arteries open. Hypovolemia (lack of enough fluid in body), hyperkalemia (elevation of the level of potassium in the blood), and kidney failure are some of the risks of taking these two groups of medication. *Beta-blockers* are a class of medications that, by dilating the arteries and relaxing the heart, may help this organ to receive better nutrition and greater oxygenation. Digoxin is an old remedy empowering the heart to pump more efficiently. As an adverse effect, beta-blockers and digoxin may seriously lower the heart rate. Judicious use of all these agents, especially in the elderly population or with individuals suffering from comorbid diseases, is highly recommended.

Obviously, the treatment of congestive heart failure is more aggressive in severe cases. Patients with end stage heart disease may need frequent hospitalization. For this group, death might be sudden.

◆   ◆   ◆

A **fall** may happen to anyone. Many falls may not even be reported to the physicians unless a serious injury occurs. The elderly may suffer from many medical conditions such as poor vision and abnormal gait. Therefore, the frequency of falls and the severity of injuries are greater among the older population as compared to the younger individuals. A fall may result in death.

The physician has to evaluate the issues of "cause and effect" of the fall, especially if there is a history of loss of consciousness. The following intriguing question has to be asked regarding a fall. "Was the fall a result of an accident or was it due to an internal medical problem, such as an irregular heart rate or low blood pressure?" A full description of how a fall occurred may help to identify the cause. A fall, due to sudden unexplained fainting, called syncope, may require hospitalization. Once the problem has been identified, the treatment must be oriented to resolve the issue. These remedies could require sophisticated medical management, such as excision of a cataract in a person with poor vision or insertion of a permanent pacemaker for the heart experiencing an irregular heart rate. On occasion, simple solutions are desired, such as using solid-sole shoes, installing a grab bar in the shower, removing a loose carpet in the bathroom, or even using hearing aids. These, and many other modalities, may prevent a slipping and, consequently, serious potential harm.

◆   ◆   ◆

One of the most common injuries after a fall is a fracture. This might occur at any age, but the frail bones of the elderly are more prone to break. The fragility of those bones is the result of a *silent* disease called **osteoporosis**. Bones are living tissues that go through breakdown and build up processes during their lifetime. In osteoporosis, there is more tear and wear of the bones rather than construction. It may take as long as 20–30 years before the bones become weak. This compromises its strength and makes it susceptible to fracture. Menopause, removal of ovaries, and long-term administration of corticosteroids are some of the risk factors associated with development of this disease. The best predictor of osteoporosis is a prior fracture. **Osteopenia** is the stage preceding the onset of osteoporosis. A bone densitometry test is a valuable method of identifying both these conditions.

Once the bone becomes osteoporotic, it may collapse or easily break. Vertebral (related to spine) collapse due to fracture is a very common phenomenon in elderly people who have not been treated for osteoporosis. Hip fracture due to a fall is another devastating problem among the same group of patients. This kind of fracture requires surgical hip replacement and long-term rehabilitation, both of which cause physical, emotional, and financial impacts. Many patients of advanced age may die after an unsuccessful hip rehabilitation process.

Prevention is the best approach to any disease. Prevention of osteoporosis has to begin in early childhood. Enough intakes of calcium and vitamin D at a younger age may prepare the groundwork for healthier bones in the future. The most common sources of calcium are dairy products (preferably low fat), eggs, fish, dried beans, and broccoli. Obtaining vitamin D is cheap because it can be produced under the skin from a moderate amount of sunlight. Taking calcium has to continue throughout our life, with higher dosages in the elderly population. This dose, usually 1000–1500 mg[9] of elemental calcium can be received either as a pill or in combination from food products. Calcium and vitamin D are equally important for prevention and treatment of osteoporosis.

Estrogen, a female hormone, and testosterone, a male hormone, are factors that produce and preserve bones. A deficiency of these hormones may cause deterioration in the strength of the bones. In such cases, hormone replacement therapy is indicated to protect the structure of the bones. A common cause of developing osteoporosis in women is menopause, due to the lack of estrogen. Preferably, the replacement of this hormone has to be initiated as soon as menopause begins and continued for many years, based upon the patient's physical condition. A routine annual mammogram is indicated for women who are treated with estrogen since this hormone may increase the risk of breast cancer. Progesterone is added to the estrogen to reduce the risk of endometrial neoplasm (cancer of the internal lining of the uterus). The combination of different types of hormone replacement therapy may also increase the risk of stroke and heart attack[20].

The regeneration of vertebral bones is feasible either with the use of an estrogen receptor modulator, called raloxifene (Evista®), which has similar effects as estrogen but with less side effects, or using a hormone, called Calcitonin, usually administered nasally.

Alendronate (Fosamax®) and risedronate (Actonel®) are two effective agents that are indicated for prevention and treatment of osteoporosis. They restore vertebral and non-vertebral bones (such as wrist or hip). Based on the doasage, these medications can be taken on a daily or weekly basis with one full glass of water at least one half-hour before a meal, preferably breakfast, and without any other medications. Ibandronate (Boniva®) is another formulation that can be taken once a month. The patient is supposed to remain in an upright position after taking these medications to prevent irritation of the lower part of the esophagus. A parathyroid by-product, called teriparatide (Fortèo®), is used for severe osteoporosis. It is self-administered as a daily injection for up to 24 months. Regardless of what medication is used to prevent or treat osteoporosis, the concomitant use of calcium and vitamin D supplement is necessary.

8

Poker Game

"…Life is like a poker game. Everyone enters this world with a different set of cards in his hands," said the sad African American man wearing a black T-shirt.

I studied him, feeling deep sorrow, and said, "That's a thoughtful view. I think I know what you are talking about!"

<u>Game 1—the glory</u>

Bernard Ferguson was a 60 years old, tall, slim African American man, with gray hair and a salt and pepper mustache. He came to my office to look for a "coach" for the games of his life. He wanted to play poker with his dearest friend and rival, "Nature"! He felt that his previous "coach doctor" was not attentive enough to make him win.

"Hello, Mr. Ferguson. How can I help you?" I asked after he sat on the chair in my exam room.

When he responded, I discovered that he stuttered, "I'm fine, doctor. The…the reason I came to see you is because I…I have blood in my urine. My physician doesn't care! He says that the bleeding is from my…my prostate cancer. He doesn't want to send me for any tests at all. I don't feel comfortable with him. That's why I came to see if you can help me," he said. Desperation was echoing in his voice.

"Did you mention prostate cancer?"

"Yes, doctor!" he explained, "But, I've already had radiation treatment for that a few years ago."

"When did your doctor send you for any follow-up tests, like an ultrasound or CAT scan of the abdomen?"

"Oh, a long time ago. Maybe a couple of years back!"

"Except for the blood in the urine, do you have any other problem?"

He smiled under his gray mustache and said sarcastically, "Doctor, do you really want to know? Well, in addition to prostate cancer, I also have diabetes, high blood pressure, and heart disease. I had a heart attack a few years ago as well. Is that enough?"

His gesture and his smile meant a lot more. It seemed like he was saying, "This life doesn't give me a break! But, I try to take it easy and the best out of it"! In reply to him, I said with a frustrated look, "That's plenty. I don't know where to start?"

"Doctor, I ain't an easy case!"

Surely, Bernard's medical problems were complex. During his examination, a strange "pulsation" in his abdomen seized my attention. When I completed my physical examination, I asked him to provide some of his urine for a test. There was indeed blood in the sample, a possible problem for patients with a history of prostate cancer. I did not feel comfortable discharging him from my office without referring him for further evaluation. In addition to some blood tests, I ordered an ultrasound of his abdomen. This appeared to me to be sufficient for an initial work-up.

"That's it, doctor?" he asked at the end of the session.

"Well, once you are done with the ultrasound, then I'd like to see you next week for a follow-up visit."

"OK, doctor, I'll see you next week."

At that time, I did not know that Bernard's routine visit would turn out to be one of the most dramatic roller-coaster medical problems that I could ever encounter. In fact, it would be like a poker game that he would play with his destiny. Nature would hold an intriguing set of cards!

Less than three days later, I received the faxed report of Bernard's abdominal ultrasound. The incidental finding was frightening and attention grabbing. My eyes widened and my heart began to pound rapidly as I read the report. "I don't know which one of us is luckier. Was it Bernard, who would need surgery as soon as possible, or I, who had ordered the ultrasound to know more about his health status?" I thought to myself. I was compelled to telephone Bernard.

"Hello, this is Dr. Tabib. I'd like to speak with Mr. Ferguson, please," I said over the phone.

"Hello, doctor. This is Mrs. Ferguson. My husband is not home now. Is there anything that I can help you with?"

"Yes, please! I need to see him. Would you ask Bernard to arrange a visit with me in the office tomorrow?"

"I'll sure do."

The next morning, Bernard appeared in my office as I expected. After he was seated in the consulting room, I said, "Mr. Ferguson, I asked you to come in earlier than our scheduled appointment because I needed to speak with you about your report."

"Did…did you find something wrong doctor?"

"Unfortunately, yes! I found a problem in your abdomen that needs a surgical intervention."

"Did…did you say sur…surgery?" he asked anxiously. "Would you explain more?"

"This doesn't have anything to do with the blood in your urine," I explained. "The bleeding could be from some scarring in your prostate as a result of previous radiation therapy! But, you have a more serious problem. The ultrasound showed that you have a big aortic aneurysm."

"Aortic aneurysm? What is this?"

"Let me make it clear. The aorta is the main artery of the body. The diameter of your aorta is 6.2 cm right now. That is almost more than double the size of a normal one. With this diameter, your aorta may rupture at any moment because of the pressure that it holds inside."

"What happens if it explodes?" he asked.

"Well! You may die!"

"Oh, boy!" Bernard had a shocked expression on his face. "What do we have to do now?"

"I'd like you to see a vascular surgeon immediately. He'll schedule you for an operation to correct the aneurysm."

"At least you are giving me some good news! The condition is correctable! When do you want me to see him?"

"Tomorrow at 10:00 A.M.!"

"How do you know the exact time?" he asked with a smile.

"Because, I've already spoken to the surgeon before you came in today. I personally made an appointment for you."

Nature definitely knew how to hide its secrets from Bernard and me. However, I was pleased to have discovered the hidden card in this game. Finding an aortic aneurysm was definitely a big surprise to both of us. Since he had multiple medical problems, he required extensive preparation before his operation. The time from the original diagnosis until the day of the surgical repair of Bernard's aortic aneurysm was less than a month. Nevertheless, during this period, I was very anxious for Bernard's safety because this large aneurysm was like a time bomb that could rupture at any moment. I was in contact with him on a weekly basis to be sure that the process of preparation would run smoothly.

Good news may come from bad news. Fortunately, Bernard's aneurysm never ruptured. It was extremely gratifying for me to know his surgery was a complete success! As I entered Bernard's room in the intensive care unit of the hospital, a day after his operation, a big smile appeared on his face. "Hello, Doc.," he said smoothly.

"Hello, Bernard! How are you feeling?" I asked enthusiastically as I held his hand.

"I've got some pain, but, hopefully, it will pass." Then, he continued as he kept a sneaky smile on his face, "Hey, doc! Do you know who came to see me today?"

"Who?"

"My former physician!"

"How did he know that you were here?"

"I don't know! But, I'll stick with you, doc!" he said and smiled with confidence.

I smiled, too, as I said, "Just get better soon. With this operation you received a gift of many more years to live. We'll continue the journey of your life together!"

That journey began with a remark. As I left Bernard's room in the hospital, a fair-skinned, beautiful young nurse with blond hair and hazel eyes approached me. She introduced herself as Bernard's personal nurse on the unit.

"Doctor, do you have any new orders for Mr. Ferguson?" she asked pleasantly.

"Only some changes in his blood pressure medications."

"OK. Just write your orders and I will follow them," she said. Then, suddenly her mood changed. A big smile appeared on her lips, her eyes gleamed, and then she commented, "It's hard to tell because he is in bed, but he looks like a tall man! Aren't his gray hair and the mustache a perfect match? Isn't he handsome?"

"Yep, you're definitely right. He is a nice guy!" I answered with a smile.

Today, many years after hearing this remark from that nurse, I still wonder, "How many times have nurses and doctors fallen in love with their patients? But, the patients never have a clue." In this case, a young, fair woman had definite feelings toward a dark-skinned man! I was wondering how much of her thoughts were sexual?

It is a glorious moment for a coach to see his player follow his guidelines and win a game proudly. Bernard was definitely a big winner in that contest with his destiny. During the hospitalization, and for many days after, my heart was filled with happiness because I had been able to prolong another human being's life. During the months following his recuperation, Bernard and his wife began to travel for pleasure, as if they were honeymooners. Finally, Bernard purchased a piece of land in Virginia for his old age and retirement. He was eager to build a house on his new property. However, as his life continued, he kept playing more games!

Game 2—the endeavor

"We just have to control this diabetes very tightly," I said to Bernard during his office visit a year after his surgery.

"What else can I do? I follow your recommendations step by step!" he said softly.

"Are you sure you take your medications as I directed?"

"Of course, doc!"

When I reviewed his treatment plan, I did not find any deviation from my recommendations in Bernard's manner of taking his medications.

"It seems that after 20 years of battling with diabetes and taking medications, now is the time to begin the insulin treatment!"

"Insulin!" he said surprisingly. "No! No! No! I do…don't wa…want to start with insulin! M…maybe you can increase m…my medications!" The anxiety made his stuttering worse!

"Your medications are in maximum dose. Your diabetes cannot be controlled anymore with these medications alone!"

"Can w…we wait a couple of more months?"

"Are you trying to bargain here with me? I know you try to take it easy. Your time is up. You can no longer escape from using insulin!"

Bernard smiled and said, "I don't want to get insulin now! I try my best with my diet. OK, Doc!"

"You are making a mistake! You leave me without choices. I'll see you in a month and, then, we'll discuss the matter further."

"No, that's too soon! I'll be back in 2 months! I have to go to Virginia in two weeks."

"Virginia? Again?"

"Doc, it's beautiful there!"

"I can't win with you. OK! You come back in two months and, then, we'll make a decision regarding your situation!"

It actually took more than six months before Bernard was ready to begin receiving the insulin shots. The training was easy and he quickly learned how to inject the insulin. He also discovered that it was not so dreadful to receive those injections. He continued with some of his oral diabetic medications at the same time. Finally, I was able to lower the level of his blood sugar with the new management. The results of those blood tests made both of us happy. As a matter of fact, Bernard was so pleased about his medical improvement that he spent most of his time in Virginia building his dream house.

Bernard was doing well for six months. Then, one early morning, Alison, his wife, paged me.

"Mrs. Ferguson! Is there anything wrong?"

"Yes! I think something is terribly wrong with Bernie," she answered with a trembling voice.

"What happened to him?"

"He...he cannot move his right arm and leg. I think he had a stroke!"

"Are you sure about what you are telling me?"

"Dr. Tabib, I'm positive."

"When did you notice the change?"

"I'm not sure. But, I think it started last night."

"OK! I think the best thing to do is to take him to the emergency room. I'd like you to call an ambulance to take him to the hospital. Can you do that?"

"Yes, yes! Of course I can do that. I'll call an ambulance immediately!"

"OK. I'll see him over there as soon as possible."

"Thank you, doctor. I'll see you soon."

In less than an hour, I was beside Bernard's bed in the emergency room. My evaluation revealed that the movement of his right extremities was limited. This indicated an acute stroke. We looked at each other, but he did not talk much. His silence in the crowded emergency room was self-explanatory. I could read the emotional pain in his eyes. The thought of being semi-paralyzed at the age of 62 was an unexpected event. His condition could prove to be a profound burden upon him and his wife.

I admitted Bernard to the hospital for further evaluation. As suggested by the consultant neurologist, we began an infusion of a blood thinner, called heparin. This was a controversial treatment considering the many hours, which had passed since the stroke occurred. I ordered a series of tests to try to reveal the reason for the stroke. Herein, began Bernard's journey in the hospital, going from floor to floor, for diagnostic assessments. Computerized tomography of his head, echocardiography, Doppler studies of the arteries going to his brain and multiple blood drawings were just part of the evaluation

Life can be cruel at times. It can definitely be surprising on other occasions as it occurred to Bernard. The next day, when I saw him in the hospital, he showed an unanticipated recovery. There was increased range of motion of his right arm and leg.

"I'm so glad to see you getting better!" I said

"Well, I'm happy, too! It is good to be able to grab things with my right hand again." Not much expression appeared on his face as he said this. It seemed he, indirectly, was informing me that we should not take our capabilities for granted because one day we might lose them.

"This is great! With some rehabilitation you are going to walk again," I said cheerfully to make the moment as happy as possible. I felt like a good coach during a successful training session of his team.

"I hope so! But I have another problem now!"

"Another problem? What is it?"

"I have bleeding from my butt when I go to the bathroom!"

"Bleeding! When did it start?"

"Since last night."

"Perhaps it is due to the heparin that you are getting. I'd better discuss this matter with the neurologist to see what we have to do next. Also, I'll ask a gastro-enterologist to come in to evaluate you. Is that OK with you?"

"All right, doctor," he answered shortly.

After I finished examining Bernard, I left his hospital room to page the neurologist. Once he answered me, we discussed Bernard's case and decided to discontinue the infusion of heparin. In the hallway, as I completed the writing of my notes in Bernard's chart, I met my colleague, Dr. John Reznick, the gastroenterologist.

"Hi, John. How are you?"

"Hi Ed. I'm fine. How is everything with you?"

"I'm OK. Listen! I have a case that might interest you. Maybe you can give me a hand."

"I'd be more than happy to help. What is this about?"

"There is a patient of mine who suffered a CVA yesterday. He also has a history of prostate cancer for which he received radiotherapy a few years ago. Since yesterday, he has been on heparin based on the consultation with the neurologist. But, the patient started bleeding from his rectum since last night. We are going to stop the heparin because of that. Now, he needs an evaluation and possibly a colonoscopy. Are you interested in getting involved in this case?" I asked.

"Sure, I'll be glad to see him today."

"Thanks a lot!" I said.

Bernard's treatment was already complicated. With the addition of the rectal bleed, his management became even more complex, requiring a colonoscopy. Early the next day, Bernard was on the table in the endoscopy unit of the hospital for evaluation of his large bowel. The stroke had made it difficult for him to roll over on the table. One of the nurses had to help him turn to the proper position.

"It will just take a minute. Start counting to ten!" the anesthesiologist said as he began injecting a medicine into Bernard's vein.

Before Bernard could finish counting to ten, the anesthetic had sedated him. After about twenty minutes, Dr. Reznick, who had performed the colonoscopy, came out of the room to write his notes. When he finished documenting his findings, he called me.

"Ed, listen. This gentleman had rectal bleed because of proctitis[1]. I cauterized some of the sites to stop the bleeding. I hope that he will be relieved from his symptoms," he explained.

"Oh! So, I guess the prior radiotherapy that he received for his prostate cancer was the cause of his proctitis!"

"Obviously, that's true. This is one of the complications of radiotherapy for this kind of cancer," he said.

I discovered that Bernard's stroke was the result of his long standing diabetes and the high blood pressure from which he suffered for many years. One stroke might be an indication of other upcoming ones. The solution to prevent another stroke in Bernard's case was either taking Aspirin or an additional medication called Clopidogrel[2] (Plavix®). Both of these medications prolong the clotting time of the blood. It sounded like a great plan. However, the reality was different. Each attempt during Bernard's hospitalization to initiate either of these treatments ended up with a heavy rectal bleed. Therefore, my colleagues and I decided not to try any further treatment with these agents. As a result, Bernard was left without any protective shield from possible future incidences. Amazingly, Bernard recuperated very well during his hospitalization. Although it was difficult, he was able to take a few steps with the aid of a walker during the last few days of his stay. When he became stable, I discharged him to a rehab facility.

---

1.   Proctitis—inflammation of the rectum, the end part of the large bowel
2.   Clopidogrel and Aspirin are platelet aggregation inhibitors

A few weeks later, after his discharge from the rehab, Bernard came into my office. His walking was fairly sable but he was forced to use a cane. As he saw me, his eyes shined, and his usual smile appeared under his mustache. His mind was sharp and he could comprehend the predicament that had hit him.

Nature, as an opponent, tried hard to defeat Bernard in this game. However, as a real winner, Bernard bounced back to continue his life. It was a tough battle for Bernard and a challenge for me. We tried to defy destiny. However, we realized we had to compromise with what Nature prepared for him. Bernard appeared to agree with that choice, too. He kept his journey through life with readiness for the next venture. After all, the house in Virginia was in the middle of construction!

Game 3—the battle

Syringes, insulin, test strips, glucometer, alcohol preps, and gauze are part of the routine daily management of every diabetic patient who requires insulin injections. So was Bernard's case. One morning, as Bernard was sitting on a chair in his kitchen, he had an argument with Alison about finding his syringes.

"Are you sure that you put your syringes here?" Alison asked Bernard while she was trying to find his syringes in the kitchen cabinets.

"I'm positive! Where else could I put them?"

"I believe you misplaced them!"

"I did not mmm…misplace them. You misplaced them!" Bernard said in a raised voice.

"Why are you getting feisty so quickly about everything?"

"I'm fine. You are the one who makes me nervous."

"I think something is wrong with you! Since the stroke four months ago, you've changed! Everything is about you…I cannot find them in this cabinet! I don't know where you hide them!" she said as she continued searching for the syringes.

"I…I haven't lost my mind. I left the…the syringes on the counter last night," Bernard said loudly.

"I don't use the insulin. You use it…Here they are! They were in the drawer," she said happily.

"How can it be? I left them on the counter! How did they get into the drawer?"

"It is very simple. They got legs!"

"Don't mess up with me woman!"

"Don't you understand jokes? OK, it's enough! Do you want me to inject your insulin or do you want to do it by yourself?"

"I'll do it! I know how to do it."

"Do you remember the dosage?" she asked nicely.

"Of course I do. It is 25 units!"

"Well, in this one you are right. I'll let you do it. Meanwhile, I'll be in the other room. If you need any help, let me know," she said and then left the kitchen.

A few minutes later, Alison heard a loud sound coming from the kitchen. She rushed there to see what had happened. As she entered the kitchen, she saw Bernard lying on the floor next to an overturned chair.

"Bernie, Bernie! Are you OK?"

"I'm fine. I just fell!" Bernard answered as he tried to rise from the floor.

"What happened?"

"I wanted to walk toward the refrigerator to pick up the insulin, but I tripped!"

"Did you get hurt?" she asked passionately.

"I don't think so!"

"I'd better make an appointment for you with the doctor. This is the second time that you have fallen this month. Something is not right with you," she said as she helped him to sit on a chair.

The next day, Bernard, accompanied by his wife, came to my office. As he walked toward me, I recognized that he was lingering more than ever. During the visit Alison commented, "He forgets things. He gets angry very easily. He already fell twice!" I noticed some gaps in Bernard's memory. I suspected he had suffered from "mini strokes" which caused his mental decline and general deterioration. At the end of the visit, I thought, "Let's try to give him Aspirin again. Maybe he can tolerate it this time without having any rectal bleed!" Therefore, I proceeded with the plan.

Unfortunately, my efforts were fruitless. Two days later, Bernard returned to my office with another episode of rectal bleeding. I was compelled to concentrate on the ongoing management of his blood pressure and diabetes to control any further damages. Yet, this attempt was also ineffective! His blood pressure fluctuated and his blood sugar did not remain stable.

One early morning, as I entered my office, the telephone rang. Bernard's wife was on the phone.

"Dr. Tabib, you have to help me!" Alison said in a panic.

"What happened, Alison?"

"Something is wrong with Bernie!" she said feverishly.

"What is it?"

"He can't talk!"

I froze in place. I thought I did not hear her well. "He can't talk! What do you mean he can't talk?"

"I mean he has not been able to talk since he got up this morning! Neither, he can move the left side of his body! He is just lying on the bed."

I felt as if I had been struck by lightening as I listened to Alison's anxious and frustrated voice. "Oh, my good Lord! He apparently had another major stroke!" I said. "Please take him immediately to the nearest hospital."

"I'll sure do!" she responded desperately.

That fateful telephone call came about one year after Bernard's first stroke. It was a dreadful picture to see him back in the hospital. As soon as he saw me, he tried to talk, but only mumbling sounds came from his mouth. He was unable to have any verbal communication at all.

"Relax, Bernard! Relax! We'll work on it until you can talk again. I'll call a speech therapist and a neurologist to help you out. Do you remember the last time you had a stroke? You eventually made it! I'm sure that you can pull through this time, too. I will try my best for you to regain the function of your left arm and leg as well. Just wait!" I said. I tried to give him some encouragement and hope, although I was not sure how much I could help him.

"Mm…hhah…ahh…ma…miff…" Bernard mumbled desperately. There was no way to understand his words.

Before I was ready to leave Bernard's room in the hospital's emergency room, I asked Alison to accompany me.

"How do you find him, doctor?" she asked as tears formed in her eyes.

"It's not good! Not good at all!"

"Do you think he can make it through?"

"I don't know! Apparently he had extensive damage to his brain. In addition to all of his troubles, he cannot eat because he might choke!"

"Oh, my gosh! This is terrible! So, how can he survive?" she asked.

"For the time being, we are going to give him some IV fluids until I can determine if he is able to swallow!"

Alison wiped the tears from her face and said, "I just hope that he will be OK!"

No matter how good a coach I wanted to be for my "team", apparently Nature was the superior player in the game. Bernard had already lost the function of his extremities and his voice. He also was not able to swallow anymore. He did not have any control of his basic needs of urination or defecation. Bernard was hit hard by his destiny this time. The struggle had become a battle for his life.

A narrow tube called nasogastric tube or NG tube was put through Bernard's nose into his stomach to administer some of his medications. I initiated an extensive management for his stroke. A neurologist, a cardiologist, and a speech therapist saw him. In addition, we had to run many diagnostic tests. The neurologist began treatment with heparin with the hopes that it would be effective this time. It definitely worked, but in an undesired way. Bernard bled again! Unfortunately, due to the heavy rectal bleedings, Bernard required three bags of blood transfusions. Finally, we had to discontinue the heparin. Hope was fading.

As I entered Bernard's room on the third day of his hospitalization, I discovered his functional right wrist was tied to the side-rail of the bed, making him completely motionless. Standing next to him were Alison and a young man.

"Hello, Dr. Tabib. This is our son, Timothy," Alison said.

"Hello, Timothy. Nice meeting you," I said as I shook his hand. I was so disturbed about Bernard's immobility that I could not finish my conversation with Timothy.

"Why is his right hand tied up?" I said as I pointed to Bernard.

"I think because he pulled out his nasal tube last night!" Alison said.

Without showing any emotions of anger or frustration, I said, "But I see that his nasal tube is in place now. Apparently, they put it back."

"Yes, the nurse explained to us that they had to reinsert the tube to give him his medications," Timothy explained.

"Well, I'm not happy that they had to tie him up." I said with dissatisfaction, "I'd better speak to the nurses!" Then, I turned to Bernard and said, "Bernie, please do not pull out your tube. This is important! This is the only way to feed you. Don't—pull out-the-tube!" Bernard nodded his head, indicating that he understood me.

When I finished my visit, Alison and Timothy accompanied me to the door.

"Doctor, do you think my dad has any chances of recovery?" Timothy asked.

"To be honest, you never know. But, he hasn't improved in the last few days. This is not a good sign."

"What are your plans for feeding him over the long term?" Alison asked.

"I'll wait for another day or two. If he still cannot swallow, we must insert a tube into his stomach directly through his abdominal wall. This is called a PEG tube, through which he will receive artificial feedings. Of course, if that's OK with you! Do you think that's what he wants us to do for him?" I asked.

"If you think that it will help him in the long run, you'd better do it," Timothy said in a sad tone.

"OK! So I'll contact one of the gastroenterologists to evaluate him for the procedure," I said.

Bernard's awareness of his surroundings and his affirmative responses to my comments gave me the impression that his cognitive functions remained appropriately intact. After I finished my conversation with the Fergusons, I approached the nursing station to find Bernard's nurse. When I located her, I said, "Why did the medical team have to give an order to tie him up to his bed? This poor guy doesn't have any function with his left arm because of the stroke. He can't even talk. And now, someone decided to put a wrist restraint on his right side, too! That's not fair to him."

"This was an order from one of the residents last night because he pulled out his NG tube," she explained.

"You can't take away the only control that is left for a him. I can't see my patient being tied up! I personally explained to Mr. Ferguson that he was not supposed to take his NG tube out. In my opinion, he understood me! I don't believe that he is going to pull it out anymore. I ask you to release the wrist restraint, please."

"Just write it down as an order!" she said.

"I'll sure do that!"

Bernard's pulling out the NG tube was an unexpected event. I was confident about the decision I had made for my patient. I hoped that with the maximum medical treatment, the nutritional supplement, and the physical therapy we could bring him back to a reasonable practical state.

In the meantime, Bernard did not regain his ability to swallow. Therefore, two days later, two gastroenterologists inserted a PEG tube. This put me at ease to be certain he could be fed properly.

Around 11:00 P.M., the night after the insertion of the PEG tube, Bernard woke up from sleep in the dark room of the hospital. Some light was penetrating through the window, giving an image of shadow to everything in the room. Bernard moved his head gently side to side. He mumbled, "…aah…haa…mm…" He felt some soreness at the tip of his penis. As he was gazing at the ceiling, he moved his right hand under the blanket and over his body. Using his instincts in seeking to comfort himself, he touched a tube and grabbed it. This was his PEG tube. As he moved the tube he felt a discomfort in his abdomen. So, he shook the tube more vigorously. All of a sudden, his PEG tube came out of his abdomen. However, the discomfort in his penis was not over. He continued searching until he felt another tube. Not knowing about the consequences of his action, he pulled the tube as forcefully as he could. Subsequently, his urinary catheter came out, too. He felt a terrible pain and started to scream.

Two nurses ran into Bernard's room when they heard him screaming. They discovered the sheets were full of blood.

"You'd better clean him up," the older nurse told the younger one. "I have to call the on-call resident. This guy needs something to calm him down. Something like Haloperidol[3]. He is out of his mind! He is crazy."

The nurse left the room to page the resident. Dr. Chang, a first year resident, answered the call.

"Dr. Chang! We have a patient here who has gone wild!" the nurse explained on the phone. "He pulled out his PEG tube and his Foley catheter! As a result, he is now bleeding! I believe that he needs some Haloperidol to calm him down! I need an order from you!"

"I can't come up now. I'm in the middle of admitting a critical patient in the emergency room," he said.

"You can come later! But, can I get an order to give him the Haloperidol?" she asked in a rushed voice.

"It sounds like he is in bad shape. OK, you can give him the Haloperidol! But..." he said.

"So, I'll write down for 2 mg!" she said.

"Would you hold on one second?" he asked. The nurse could hear him on the phone discussing the issue with someone else. Then, the resident said, "OK, my senior resident agrees with the dose. Do you need me to come for reinsertion of the Foley?" he asked.

"Don't worry about the Foley. I'll take care of it for you. But, come in later to evaluate him. If he continues to bleed I'll call you back," she said.

Bernard had some irritation at the tip of his penis, which he did not know how to ease. The lack of verbal communication made it difficult for him to convey his feelings to other people. Bernard, the champion in two rounds of a poker game with Nature, was already disabled by his incompetent mental status due to the stroke. Now, after receiving the Haloperidol, he was completely knocked down.

During the next few days after the incidence, while Bernard spent many hours sleeping, he received his food and medications through a brand new PEG tube. Unfortunately, the staff was forced to put the wrist restraint on from time to time to prevent him from causing any more unpredicted accidents. As he was weaned off the sedative medications, he regained some of his consciousness, making it possible to be discharged. Then, in order to continue my care for him, I ordered his transfer to a rehabilitation center with which I was affiliated.

---

3.   Haloperidol—a psychotropic medication with sedating activity.

Against all my expectations, Bernard became more aware of his environment. He kept having the smile under his mustache every time I saw him in the rehab center. Yet, I had my doubts that he ever really recognized me after he was placed in that facility. Sadly, his voice never returned, making him unable to communicate with me or anybody else verbally.

Ten days later, as I was doing my daily round in the rehab center, I received a call from Bernard's nurse. "Dr. Tabib! You'd better come to see your patient, Mr. Ferguson. He's throwing up and acting bizarre! There is something wrong with him!" she said.

When I visited Bernard, he appeared very agitated. He was moving his head from side to side with occasional short pauses in order to look at me. I knew one of the complications of having a PEG tube was occasional vomiting. My evaluation revealed that his problem might be more intricate.

An hour later, Bernard was back in the hospital, where he deteriorated rapidly. During the next few days, hopes were completely fading away for any recovery. Eventually, I found the right time to speak with his family during the end of one of my visits. Alison, Timothy and Bernard's older brother, Michael, were all at his bedside.

"He gets recurrent strokes. These affect his memory and his mental status. He is too sick to pull through!" I explained to them.

"He is just lying down and doing nothing! There is absolutely no communication! He is not able to eat and he cannot control his bodily functions at all!" Michael commented with frustration.

"Well, you are right. Unfortunately that's the story of end of life. At this point, we can either provide comfort care or keep him alive by supplying him with artificial nutrition through the tube," I explained.

"So, do you think that any further treatment is futile?" Timothy asked.

"That's what I believe. But, still, the choice is yours," I answered.

"Dr. Tabib! I think the time has come," Alison said. "We better stop the treatments."

"Let me ask you this question. How are you planning to do that doctor, if we let him go?" Michael asked.

"I have to minimize his nutrition and give him some morphine for comfort. The rest is in the hands of Mother Nature...Is that OK with you?" I questioned.

Suddenly, silence filled the atmosphere momentarily until Alison broke it. "I think we're all in agreement with that plan. We already had a feeling that this was coming soon. He has suffered enough! I lived with him for so many years. I know that he never wanted to be in this shape."

"Do you know how long it will take until he passes away?" Michael asked.

"You never know. But, it usually takes about 3 to 7 days!" I answered.

Throughout my conversation with the Fergusons, I tried to support them in their decision. I showed a strong veneer as I discussed Bernard's destiny, but my heart was breaking. I knew they were in pain. I talked to them about the life and death of a patient, a human being, whom I had taken care of for three years. At this time, Bernard was playing his final show on the stage of life. As I made my departure from the hospital, I left a family in despair. Then, I had to deal with my own emotional state of separation from a patient. As I sat in my car, this feeling overwhelmed me. I covered my eyes with my hands trying to find a moment to pray for Bernard.

Everyday, I went to visit Bernard in the hospital after initiation of the treatment called "comfort care". Against all my previous experiences, he did not die in three days, or seven days, or even ten days! Maybe, he was trying to tell me that he was still the winner in his game with destiny. He kept living and I had to increase the dose of morphine. It was heartbreaking to see him dying, but I knew there was no other choice. On the fourteenth day into the comfort care, I entered Bernard's room. Michael, a devoted brother, was sitting at the end of Bernard's bed. He was wearing a black T-shirt. He was looking at Bernard quietly.

"Hello, doctor," he said when he saw me.

"Hello, Michael."

"He just doesn't want to die," he said calmly but with profound sadness.

The atmosphere of the room was filled with a heavy grief. I found myself unable to respond to Michael. I nodded my head and passed in front of him to get closer to Bernard. His face was serene, like an angel, and his body was motionless, in peace. I performed my routine examination and then stood quietly next to his bed.

"You know, doctor," Michael said, "life is like a poker game. Everyone enters this world with a different set of cards in his hands."

"That's a thoughtful view. I think I know what you are talking about!" I said. I stayed in the room for a few more moments and then I left after a farewell to Michael. Bernard, amazingly, stayed alive long enough so I could hear this splendid comment from his brother.

That same night, Bernard passed away!

◆   ◆   ◆

The scope of Bernard's medical problems was certainly a challenge for me. Throughout my medical career, I have seen many patients who passed away during the comfort care. In this regard, however, Bernard surpassed any one of them. He was indeed a true winner. He finished his last game with Nature at the age of sixty-three. I still miss his gestures, his troubled voice, and even his lingering walk after his first stroke. Bernard died due to the complications of long-term diabetes, hypertension, and the consequences of the treatment for his prostate cancer. I blame his death mostly upon his long-term uncontrolled diabetes. He had suffered form diabetes for many years, long before he was under my care!

These days, I provide medical care for Alison. She often travels to the state of Virginia to take care of her land. She is also playing a poker game with Nature to discover her destiny. How strange can fate be? She suffers from diabetes, too!

MEDICAL WISDOM

Imagine what happens to a piece of unpainted metal when it is left outside. After a few weeks, the air and the rain make it rusty and unusable. This process is comparable to the decay of the internal linings of vessel walls due to silent diseases. Early stages of **diabetes**, elevated blood pressure (**hypertension**), and high cholesterol (**hypercholesterolemia**) do not cause any pain or other symptoms. Unlike the decay process of the piece of metal in a few weeks, the biological deterioration of the blood vessels due to the adverse effects of those diseases takes many years. The final outcome of this corrosion would be devastating if these diseases progressed for many

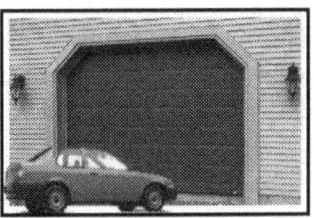

Figure 1- Sugar molecules go into the cells, like a car entering a garage

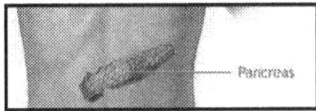

Figure 2 – Pancreas is located in the upper part of the abdomen

years without adequate control. The treatment to minimize the extent of the damage must be initiated as soon as the diagnosis is established.

A remote control, with fresh batteries, may help you open your garage door from a distance. A sensor behind the garage door is needed to receive the radio-wave signals emitted by the remote control. Old batteries in the remote control or malfunction of the garage door-sensor will not let the door to open (figure 1). In our body, a similar mechanism occurs during the absorption of sugar molecules. As food enters the intestine, it breaks down into small molecules of sugar that are able to be absorbed into the blood stream. These molecules trigger the release of a hormone from the pancreas (figure 2). This hormone, called *insulin*, acts like a remote control to enable the sugar molecules to enter the tissues. Insulin activates a sensor, called a *"receptor"*, located on the cell. It facilitates the entrance of the sugar into the tissues.

A gradual depletion of insulin causes an elevation of the sugar in the blood (hyperglycemia). Many factors, such as genetic factors, obesity, some medications, a non-healthy diet, or lack of exercise may contribute to the reduction of the insulin level. The worsening of the hyperglycemia causes a disease called diabetes.

Diabetes is commonly divided into two categories depending on the age of onset and the development, or the pathophysiology, of the disease. Type-I, frequently called juvenile diabetes, starts at a younger age, as early as childhood. In this type, the pancreas lacks the ability to produce insulin. Type-II, or adult onset diabetes, begins later in life. In this case, the pancreas initially tries to offset the high levels of sugar by releasing larger amounts of insulin into the blood stream. As the compensation fails over years, the production of insulin diminishes and eventually fades completely. Over the years, a malfunction develops in the insulin receptors in the tissues, causing them to be resistant to the hormone. This results in the increase of the level of sugar in the blood. In other terms, once the sensor of the garage door has lost its sensitivity, it does not matter whether the remote control works properly or not; your car will remain outside.

In the beginning, diabetes presents itself with increased thirst, hunger, and urination. Later, as the blood vessels, especially the smaller ones, become "rusted" by the elevated blood sugar, different tissues and organs are endangered of mal-functioning. These organs are called "target" organs. The most important ones are the brain, the eyes, the kidneys, and the heart. Stroke, blindness, kidney fail-ure, or heart attacks are some of the complications, which might develop after many years of suffering from uncontrolled diabetes. Patients with diabetes may experience numbness of the fingers or toes, feel nauseous, or even occasionally vomit. Diabetic men may become impotent, a problem which results in emo-tional consequences.

With Type I diabetes, the main treatment is administration of insulin. In Type II diabetes, depending upon the progression of the disease, diet, medica-tions, insulin, or a combination of these methods may be used for management.

Some medications, such as *Acarbose* or *Miglitol*, delay the absorption of sugar from the intestine. *Sulfonylureas* are very common medications used in early Type II diabetes. They have the dual action of inducing the release of more insulin from the pancreas and increasing the sensitivity of different tissues to insulin. The liver is an organ that may produce sugar in our body. An agent, called *Metformin*, reduces this production and increases the tissue sensitivity to insulin. Newer agents, such as *Thiazolidinediones*, fight against the insulin resistant tissues caused by diabetes. *Insulin* is marketed in different types based on its onset and duration of action. This agent can be injected either into the skin or administered intrave-nously. Research is underway for administration of insulin through inhalation. All of these agents may develop side effects that require close follow-up by a phy-sician.

The challenges of diabetes and its complications do not end with controlling blood sugar. Many diabetic patients may have elevated cholesterol and blood pressure, as well. New guidelines from the third report of the National Choles-terol Education Program consider diabetes a coronary heart disease risk equiva-lent[10]. It is recommended that the cholesterol level of diabetic patients be reduced as low as the levels of patients with heart disease. This strategy signifies the importance of management of hypercholesterolemia in this group. Controlling other risk factors such as smoking, obesity, and hypertension, aids in the reduction of complications from this disease.

◆   ◆   ◆

An **aneurysm** is the enlargement of the diameter of an artery and the weakening of its wall. Once this occurs, the pressure inside the artery may lead to its rupture. This is similar to the bursting of an over-inflated balloon. The result is a severe bleeding with ominous consequences.

The aorta is the largest artery originating from the heart. It runs through the chest and in the back of the abdomen to distribute blood to every organ system. A rupture of the aorta, for any reason, may lead to massive bleeding and probably death. A small number of the elderly population may develop an aneurysm of the aorta in the abdomen, called an "**abdominal aortic aneurysm**". This is the most dangerous aneurysm in the body. If the diameter of the aorta with an aneurysm exceeds 6 cm, it is called a large aneurysm. It has a high possibility of rupture. As the aneurysm grows, the risk of rupture increases as well. The treatment for an aneurysm is a surgical intervention and replacement with a synthetic graft. The long-term survival of these patients is determined by the presence or absence of diseases in other vascular beds, which may lead to myocardial infarction and stroke—the principal causes of death[11].

◆   ◆   ◆

I know life is precious. Yet, I don't know if destiny is like poker, soccer, chess, or any other games. All we do is to play a game with a superpower, called Nature. We win many times, however it will show its lead in the final game. We better enjoy the game before it is over!

9

Puzzle of a Mysterious Infection

Rachel was a fifty-five year-old, very gentle, quiet, diminutive woman. She walked into my office for the first time on a rainy afternoon. After a brief introduction in the waiting room, I asked her to come to the exam room. Her main problem was a cough. She made her inquiries in a respectful manner indicating she was apprehensive. Her uncertainty about my answers echoed in her voice in every step of our conversation. As part of taking her history, I learned that her married daughter was going to college, so Rachel was very busy helping to raise her grandchild. During my examination, I discovered her blood pressure was high, and it remained high even at the end of the session when I rechecked it. After giving a prescription for her cough, I asked her to return for a follow-up visit.

I established a very close relationship with Rachel and her daughter, Katherine during the following year. She continued to come in for her regular check-ups and especially for her blood pressure problem. She eventually began taking a blood pressure pill. She was always compliant with her medication. But, she never complained of any other significant symptoms.

One summer day, I received an urgent call from Katherine.

"Doctor, mom is having a severe left-sided chest pain", she said.

The first thing that went through my mind was that Rachel was having a heart attack!" How long has she been having pain?" I asked

"For 3 days! She is running a temperature, too!"

Her answer put me at ease. "Does she have any shortness of breath?"

"No." She responded.

"Does the pain radiate to any other area?" I inquired.

"No!"

"Would you like to bring her in for an evaluation?"

"Yes! Is it possible to see her today?"

"Sure!" I replied. I suggested that she come in as soon as she could.

Less than half an hour later Rachel was sitting in front of me in the exam room accompanied by Katherine. Rachel, as usual, was so calm that at first glance, I did not believe she was in any distress. She tried, in a low tone of voice, to explain to me that her problem may not be serious! She complained of a pain that was in the left side of her chest. Any movement of her chest increased her pain. Without any further questions, I asked her to allow me to examine her chest. To my surprise, there was a big area of redness on her left breast, which must have been painful! Surprisingly, Rachel showed a very high threshold for pain. There was no doubt in my mind that she was suffering from a serious infection. She had a condition called mastitis, an infection of the breast. This was not a matter I could treat without hospitalization. After a brief discussion, I asked her to go to the nearest hospital for further treatment. My request was not without resistance!

"Doctor, do you really think that I have to go to the hospital?" she asked. "Can't you give me an antibiotic? I will be back tomorrow for follow-up."

I looked away and started to nod my head as a sign of negative response. I glanced at her daughter for a moment, and then I looked at Rachel. Her eyes were begging me not to send her to the hospital.

"Rachel, I am afraid you are going to be in trouble if you decide to stay out of the hospital. In my opinion it is not worth trying. By staying home you may become more ill. You'd better listen to me!" I showed firmness in my decision.

"OK," Rachel said as if she has been defeated in a battle.

Two hours later I was on my way to visit Rachel in the emergency room. I knew that this kind of infection could not develop without an underlying disease. During the drive to the hospital, I kept trying to think of the reason why she had the infection, "Maybe she has cancer! But, she had a mammography 6 months ago that was completely normal. What else could be wrong?"

It was 6 PM when I arrived at the very busy emergency room. I found Rachel, waiting along with Katherine in one of the corner beds. "Doctor! If this is cancer, please let me know! I want to be prepared," she said sadly when I encountered her. It seemed she was reading my mind. "Rachel, first let's treat the infection and then we will discuss the other issues." I avoided answering her directly.

After my initial evaluation, I discussed the case with one of the infectious disease consultants. We agreed to call in a surgeon to further explore the problem. Rachel definitely needed to remain hospitalized to receive the appropriate treatment.

This time as in the past I turned to Dr. John Montgomery to evaluate Rachel. It was not long before Dr. Montgomery arrived in the emergency room.

"Hi, John." I said.

"Hi, Ed. What's up?" asked Dr. Montgomery.

"I have this nice lady. She's got mastitis of her left breast. She definitely needs antibiotics. However, we were thinking that she might need more work-up."

"Well, let me take a look."

While Dr. Montgomery was evaluating Rachel, I started to write my notes. It was not long before he came back. "I have to poke in a needle!" he said. I had guessed that to identify the bacteria he would be interested in taking a culture from the area of infection by using a syringe to aspirate some pus. It is always important to know your enemy before an attack! I agreed with his decision. I approached Rachel to explain about the procedure. After a short discussion she realized that we were talking about inserting a needle into her breast. She agreed with the procedure. Shortly, Dr. Montgomery appeared with his surgical tray. I went back to finish my notes.

Before I finished writing two sentences, Dr. Montgomery was back.

"Hey, this was quick!" I said.

"I didn't get anything. Not even a worthy piece. I have to open her up! It looks like she has an abscess!" he said.

"With this pace of yours I believe you are planning to do a surgery on her. So, when are you gonna do the surgery? Is this going to be tonight?"

"Yep! I don't like to postpone these things."

"Please remember to take a biopsy. You know! It might be cancer!"

"I won't forget. This will definitely be done!"

After a brief farewell, he left the emergency room. I walked down to Rachel's corner space to notify her about our decision.

"Rachel, you need to have a surgery done." I explained.

"Doc! Do you think it is necessary to go through this? If there is something going on, please, let me know!" Rachel said.

"Listen, Rachel, I still don't know what is going on with you! But, I know that your condition is serious enough to require surgery."

Rachel suddenly became quiet. She definitely appeared frightened.

"Rachel! To get to the bottom of this, I ask you to be patient and cooperative." I said.

She nodded her head as a sign of agreement.

For some patients, it might take a long time to establish trust in physician. Rachel was one of those individuals. I had known Rachel for almost a year. In most instances, before making any decision, she showed plenty of hesitancy. However, this was the first time I felt she demonstrated confidence in my guidance. As I left the hospital, I felt certain about my decision, but uncomfortable, knowing that Rachel did not want to be there. Now, she was facing an inevitable surgical procedure that she had never contemplated.

Meanwhile, Rachel's daughter left the hospital to return home to take care of her baby. Rachel remained in the emergency room. The nurse began the intravenous antibiotic that Dr. Montgomery had ordered. Rachel felt cold and asked for an extra blanket. A feeling of loneliness and seclusion started to rise in her heart. She grasped the blanket and squeezed it, seeking comfort. She was terribly afraid of having cancer of the breast. This thought would not allow her to rest.

It was around one o'clock in the morning when Rachel was taken to the operating room. Her heart was pounding from anxiety of an unknown journey. This was the first time in her life that she had to have surgery. She saw Dr. Montgomery in the corner of the operating room, talking to a nurse. Before she could figure out what was going on she was in a deep sleep.

The day after the surgery I went to visit Rachel. On my way to her room, I met Dr. Montgomery in the hallway. I was prepared to hear that Rachel had breast cancer. However, the news was just the opposite of what I anticipated. "I could not see any obvious sign of cancer!" he said. This made me very happy, but it did not solve the puzzle of how Rachel developed that infection in her breast.

I found Rachel's room on the third floor of the hospital. It was a nice, quiet room. She looked very happy when she saw me. I showed interest in her progress. She was pleased that the worst was over. Being curious about her condition I asked her an open question, "Rachel, did you ever notice any abnormal finding in your breast?"

"No!" she answered. Then after a brief pause she said, "Nothing, except a little milk that came out of my breasts from time to time. For example, this happened when I was having a mammography!"

Playing a medical detective, I thought I might have discovered the first clue. "How long have you had this problem?" I asked.

Her answer was astonishing. "About 20 years!" she said calmly.

"Twenty years! And you never told me that!"

"But, doctor, this is something normal to me! I have always had it since the birth of my last child!"

"Do you call this normal? Now, you are talking. Finally! Finally, I think I know what is going on with you!"

As I left Rachel's room, I knew that half the puzzle was solved. She had a condition called *galactorrhea*. I ordered a series of tests for further work-up. I was anxious to receive the reports as soon as possible. However, Rachel was discharged from the hospital before I could obtain the results. So, in a telephone conversation, I asked her to make an appointment with me in a few days. I was confident I could direct her down the right path to solve her condition.

◆   ◆   ◆

One week passed before Rachel showed up in my office. She looked happy. As we engaged in conversation regarding her condition, she asked, "Doctor, did you find out what was wrong with me?"

"Well! I found some abnormalities in the blood test. The results may shock you! But, they are not really as bad as they seem."

"It doesn't sound good. I know! I have no choice other than to listen to you!"

"I'm telling you. It just may sound scary, but we have to deal with it."

"OK, doctor! I'm ready."

"Rachel, I believe you have a brain tumor!"

Silence was her answer. Rachel did not utter a word after I broke the news to her. She bowed her head for a moment and then very slowly looked up at my eyes. Then, she said, "Doctor! You could tell me anything except this! And, you are telling me that this is not bad news!"

"No, Rachel! It is possible to take care of this. Sometimes, even a medication may help." Then I continued, "Well I have to add. If you don't take care of this, you may end up being blind!"

"Please, doctor! I don't want to hear about this any more! I don't want to hear about the possibility of having a brain tumor at all! Please, I also ask you not to mention this to my daughter!"

Rachel understood the nature of her medical problem, but she was in denial. That is a common phase in accepting the bad outcome of a test. As I discussed the matter with her, I kept my voice calm and extremely serene. Deep inside myself, I wished I could grab her arms, shake her and tell her, "Rachel, wake up! Without intervention, you'll become blind! Stop denying your problem! You need an urgent treatment!" But, my hands were bound by my professional morality. The key for adequate and appropriate management is to persuade and encourage the patient to take steps toward the treatment, rather than to raise fears of disability. Rachel went home and did not discuss her news with anyone. As a matter of fact, she did not return for her follow-up appointment the next week.

Further testing was essential for a final diagnosis in Rachel's case. How could I convince her to go for the additional testing? I called and requested that she come in for more evaluation. However, each time she had an excuse for not returning to my office. The main excuse was that she had to take care of her grandson. I realized she was not ready to talk to me or any other physician about her condition. The most mysterious secret in her story was why she did not want to hear anything about a brain tumor?

◆   ◆   ◆

One month later, Rachel finally showed up in my office, accompanied by Katherine. I sensed that Rachel had spoken about her medical problem to her daughter. She appeared calm as always. During our conversation, her head was down and she made minimal eye contact. I recognized some signs of a depressive mood. She was not in a mood to talk. But, I was eager to help her.

"Rachel, let's talk about your situation," I commented. "What is your understanding of a brain tumor?"

Finally, this question nailed down the last piece of the puzzle. The answer was definitely surprising. "You know, doctor! This was not happy news for me. My mother had a brain tumor. She died from it!"

In this instance, it was my turn to remain quiet. I did not know how to answer her. I realized that her fears concerned death and not blindness. I shook my head and I explained, "But, your circumstance might be different."

"Do you really think so?"

"Of course! We have to do more tests to evaluate your condition. A CAT scan of your head might be sufficient to give us more information."

"Do you believe this will give you a proper answer?"

"We definitely can try it."

"Do you really think that my problem can be solved?"

"Well! It is highly possible. Let's not give up hope!"

"OK, doctor! I am ready to give it a try."

A ray of optimism was also established in my communication with Rachel and my management of her problem.

This was the first time Rachel was ready to take action. Just one week after our conversation the CAT scan report of her head was on my desk. My initial hypothesis was correct. The results of the blood test and the CAT scan were consistent with her having a tumor in the hypophysis, the lowest part of her brain. A hypophyseal tumor may result in galactorrhea. It was the accumulation of the milk in her breast which caused the infection and the formation of an abscess. Fortunately, this was probably a curable disease. As I learned those facts, I called her.

"Listen! I was right about my presumptive diagnosis. You indeed have a brain tumor!" I said.

"So, do you think that I need surgery for that, too?"

"Not really! Your fears are in vain! You just have to take a medication to shrink the tumor."

"Is it that easy?"

"I told you it just sounded terrible, but it is not!"

"Where do I go from here?"

"I will refer you to an endocrinologist for follow-up."

"Are you telling me that I will stay alive?"

"Didn't you tell me that your daughter needs you so she can continue her education? So, you got it!"

"Doctor! I don't know how to thank you."

"I'm happy you will be safe."

◆   ◆   ◆

Less than a month later I had a telephone call from Rachel. She informed me about the report of a new CAT scan of her head, which had been ordered by the endocrinologist. This one showed a remarkable shrinkage of the tumor! Rachel could not have been happier. She must, however, continue taking medication for the rest of her life.

MEDICAL WISDOM

The hypophysis is the gland that regulates many of the functions of other glands in our body. It is located under the intersection of the optic nerves. These nerves connect the eyes to the brain. An enlargement, called **hypophyseal tumor**, may push those nerves upward and cause blindness.

Prolactin is one of the hormones which are produced from the hypophysis. Production of prolactin stimulates the production of milk from the breasts. This happens most frequently right after pregnancy. An excess production of prolactin beyond a certain period of time after giving birth is abnormal. This might happen with frequent stimulation of the breasts, for example during sexual relations. Another reason could be an over-secretion of prolactin from the hypophysis because of a tumor. In the early stages of this disease, a medication, such as Bromocriptine, may shrink the tumor and avert blindness. In advanced cases, the patient may need a surgical procedure. Rachel was lucky to have a small tumor.

The author suggests that radiologists and radiology technicians inform the primary physicians in cases of the extraction of a milky discharge from the nipples of a patient during a mammography. This may help in the early diagnosis of hypophyseal tumors due to an excess production of prolactin.

◆　　　◆　　　◆

When you discover a lump or another change in your breast, it is important to know what it is. It is normal to be alarmed. However, you have reasons to be reassured. Most women, at some time in their lives, develop lumps in their breasts. Most lumps are *not* cancerous. In fact, 8 of 10 lumps are harmless. To be sure that a lump or other changes is not breast cancer, you need to have some portion or the entire lump removed (a biopsy). A diagnosis can be made by looking at the cells under a microscope to establish the nature of the tissue to be either normal or cancerous.

Breast cancer is the most common cancer diagnosed in women today. It even occurs in a small number of men. In the United States, close to 200,000 women are diagnosed with breast cancer each year. Adults, in all ages and races, are affected: 1 in 9 whites, 1 in 11 African-Americans, and 1 in 20 Hispanic and Asian women will develop breast cancer during their lifetime. Nobody knows for certain why some women develop breast cancer and others do not. Age and some genetic factors may play a role in this process. Therefore, having an initial mammography in early age for women with a strong family history, and for the rest of women at the age of 40, is essential. Thereafter, an annual mammogram is recommended.

The treatment for breast cancer is surgery, radiation, chemotherapy, or a combination of these. These treatments are chosen based on the progression of the disease. The remedy can be as simple as a lumpectomy, in which the breast cancer, a little normal breast tissue around the lump, and some lymph nodes under the arm are removed. On the other hand, it can be as complicated as surgical removal of one or both breasts (mastectomy). Based on the nature of the cancerous tissue, a hormone blocker, such as tamoxifen (Nolvadex®) is given orally to prevent any further growth of the cancer. Breast reconstruction or surgery to rebuild a breast is a routine option for any woman who has lost a breast because of cancer.

Emotional instability might follow the diagnosis of breast cancer. To cope with these feelings, survivors of breast cancer are recommended to share their thoughts with their friends, family members, other breast cancer survivors or support groups. These patients are also encouraged to use biofeedback, meditation, yoga, and avoid stress to possibly boost their immune system and prolong their lives. To obtain valuable information, some contact telephone numbers are listed at the end of this book.

10

A Clean Bill of Health

"Hello, Mrs. Abramov. I haven't seen you in a long time!" I said.

"Hello, Doctor. Well, I was not able to visit you because my previous health insurance coverage was very problematic. Now, I have Medicare! I understand that is OK," she said.

"You were always welcome in my office, regardless of your coverage. I'm glad you are back here!"

Monir Abramov was a Middle Eastern sixty-five years old patient of mine, whom I had known for a long time. She was a short and mildly obese woman. Her gray hair was silky but never groomed. She always wore multiple layers of cloths, a typical grandmother style, as if it was never-ending winter! She would visit me from time to time to receive treatment for her high blood pressure, high cholesterol, asthma, and not to forget, the calluses on her feet. Her last visit had been six months ago. One mid spring day, her daughter-in-law, Jasmine, a trim and neat young lady with auburn colored hair, brought her to my office for a routine follow-up visit.

"Doctor, you know how much I love you! You are my light in the dark. You are my hope. I wish you would stay forever. The Lord should help you to help the weak!" Monir said.

I could not stop laughing in my heart after hearing her. It sounded as if she was praying rather than talking to me! But, who was I not to accept such wonderful phrases? Of course, this amiability was a pleasant new beginning for taking care of her. I believed she had returned to be followed by me because of the compassion I extended for her feelings and an understanding of her medical problems.

Monir had a gentle spirit. Her weakness was the fear of the unknown, a very common characteristic of many of us. My examination began only after we concluded a discussion about the past. When I asked about her medications, I discovered another physician had changed them to some extent. My evaluation revealed high blood pressure, which required the addition of a medication to her existing therapeutic regimen.

"Listen! I think you have to take this new medication to regulate your blood pressure. Here is your prescription." As I handed her the prescription I said, "I'll see you in two weeks for a follow-up visit."

"Doctor, I'm really nervous. Do you think I will be OK? You know I've had this blood pressure for a long time. I'm afraid that I might have a stroke! This is scary to me. I'm getting old, but I don't want to be a burden to my children. Please, help me! Please!"

"You worry too much! Let me see you again in two weeks to find out more about your blood pressure. If we control it well enough, we'll certainly reduce the risks of having a stroke."

It is a very common reaction for elderly people to think about the possible deterioration of their functional capacity. This may cause them to be anxious and worried about their future. They may perceive their personal physician as someone with a superior power to relive their fears and apprehension. Giving reassurance to those patients may have positive effects on their lives. Close follow up also is an additional way for reinforcement. That was what I did for Mrs. Abramov.

Two weeks later, Mrs. Abramov returned for a follow-up visit. Her anxiety level was almost unchanged. She was still worried about her future.

"Mrs. Abramov, your blood pressure is much better now. I'm very glad we could finally bring it under control. Isn't that good news?" I asked.

"Doctor Tabib, are you serious? Is my blood pressure really improved? Are you sure about it? You know! I have children and grandchildren. The little kids and their parents still need me to help them. I want to be around to see them. They work, work and work. You know how difficult it is to make a living in this country! I don't want to be crippled! I don't want them to take care of me."

"I'm telling you the truth! You're doing just fine! I also received the results of your recent blood tests. It shows the level of your cholesterol is excellent. I don't think there is anything to be worried about at all!"

"God bless you! So you mean that I am not going to have any stroke?"

"Stroke? I don't understand why you have to think about a stroke. You are in a good shape. You are far from becoming disabled. Please, calm down! Just remember to take your medications as I recommended."

"This is good news. I'm so sorry to put you through all this trouble, doctor. So, I should continue with the same treatment until I see you again?"

"That's right. I'll see you again for follow-up in less than a month."

Before she left the exam room, she shocked me again by repeating her question. She turned toward me and asked, "So, you are telling me that I'm OK and I'm not supposed to be worried! Is that correct?"

"Mrs. Abramov! I truly believe you are in a stable condition with these medications. I don't see any reason to worry. Try to relax!"

"Thank you, doctor. I'll see you in less than a month," she said. Then, she embraced me, giving me a hug and kissed me on the cheek.

I was so glad to make Monir confident about her medical condition. I believed I used both medicine and its art to make her content. The state of my mind also had been calmed because I felt her medical problems were completely under control. I sent her home in a good mood. I was eager to see her in a month for follow up.

Two days later

Two days after Monir had visited me in the office, Jasmine telephoned her. "Mom!" Jasmine said, "I have to ask you a big favor! My baby sitter called in sick today. I have a lot of things to do. I must go shopping. I also have an appointment with the dentist. I cannot take Jonathan with me. It is going to be too much if I have to take him along! Could you possibly come to my home to take care of the baby, please?"

"It will be my pleasure to be there. I love you just like one of my own children. It's no problem for me to help you out," Monir replied.

"Thank you. I really appreciate it. So, I'll come now to pick you up."

"I'll wait for you."

Shortly thereafter, Jasmine picked up Monir. While driving back, the two women talked about many subjects. It did not take long before they reached Jasmine's house. As they entered the house, Jasmine said, "By the way, I forgot to ask you about your doctor's visit! I'm sorry that I couldn't take you there last time."

"That's OK! I know how busy you are at times. I took the bus. The doctor said that I was in very good shape. He also said I was too worried about my condition!"

"I'm glad to hear that. Are you still on the same medications?"

"Yes. This time he did not change any of them!"

"Well. That's good. Did you bring your medicines with you so you can take them while you are here?"

"I know that I'm getting old, but my memory still is working! Of course I brought them with me," Monir said.

"OK, just be sure that Jonathan does not reach them. He is only two and a half years old! He picks up everything and puts it in his mouth. Watch him carefully!"

"This is not my first time taking care of him. Nevertheless, I will be very cautious."

"Thank you for your understanding. All right, I have to leave now! You know where Jonathan's food is. I think it would be fine if you want to give him his meal now. It's his lunchtime. By the way, just as a reminder, the number of my cellular phone is on the refrigerator. If you have any questions, just give me a buzz!" Jasmine said as she was leaving the house.

"Don't worry at all. Everything will be fine."

After Jasmine left the house, Monir lifted and kissed Jonathan.

"Mama, mama, play!" Jonathan said.

"We'll play. We are gonna have a lot of fun together today. But, let's go to the kitchen and have some food first. You must be hungry."

Monir put Jonathan down and walked into the kitchen.

Robin, Monir's son, was a robust, tall man with large brownish eyes and scarce amount of hair on his head. He was busy behind his desk at work. Since he knew his mother would be at his house caring for his son, he decided to take a moment to call and see how everything was going. The telephone rang several times, but no one answered. He hung up and continued with his work. Half an hour later, he tried again. Still, there was no answer at his house. So he called his wife on the cellular phone. He hoped Jasmine could tell him what had happened.

"Jasmine? Where are you now?" Robin asked.

"I'm in the dental office. Is anything wrong?"

"Listen! No one answers the phone at home. Did you pick up my mom to take care of Jonathan?" Robin asked.

"Of course, I did. I brought her in personally."

"So, why is there no answer at home?"

"Don't worry! Probably she is in the backyard playing with Jonathan. Call her up in half an hour. She'll be back in the house by then."

In less than half an hour, Jasmine decided to call home to speak with Monir and ask how things were going. However, there was still no response. She began to worry and called Robin.

"Robin, you're right! She doesn't answer! I am worried! That is not typical of her. She always answers the telephone calls."

"What time did you bring her in?"

"Around 12 o'clock."

"Now, it is way past one o'clock. Where is she? Do you think there might be something wrong?"

"I hope you are mistaken. But, the whole thing makes me nervous!"

"You know what! It's more than an hour that she's in the house! She is supposed to be there. I'm troubled. Something may have happened to her or to Jonathan. You call the police to go over there! I'll leave work now and go home to see what has happened!"

"OK, Robin. I'll be there as soon as possible!" she said anxiously.

As Robin arrived at his home, he saw that a police car was already parked in the front. The officer was at the door, ringing the bell.

"Sir, my name is Robin. I live here," Robin explained to the officer as he approached the entrance door of his house.

"Oh! It's good to see you. I almost wanted to break in. I hear a baby crying inside, but no one came to the door," the officer said.

"Oh, my gosh! That has to be my son! Let me open the door!" he said, as he tried to find his house key. His hands were shaking and his face felt flushed as he tried to unlock the door. As he entered the house, Jonathan ran toward him.

"Daddy! Daddy!" Jonathan cried.

Jonathan's face was streaked with tears. Robin hugged him to calm him down. The officer was standing behind Robin.

"He is probably frightened. Your wife left a message that your mom was supposed to take care of him. So, where is she?" the officer asked.

"I don't know! That is not like my mom! She is usually a responsible person!" he answered. Then, he started to call out, "Mom, mom…Are you here?" There was no reply.

Robin and the officer began to search for his mother. Robin entered the kitchen. The scene that he found shocked him. Monir was lying on the floor, unconscious. Her eyes were closed and she appeared pale. The floor around her head was covered with a pool of blood, indicating a severe impact. The lower part of her clothes was wet from urine.

Robin put Jonathan down. He rushed over to check his mother. "Mom! Mom! Are you OK?" he said. Monir did not respond. "Oh, my Lord! Is she dead?" Robin asked.

"Don't panic! Let's check first if she is breathing!" the officer said as he entered to the kitchen. Then, he brought his head close to Monir's face. "Yes, she's breathing! Let me check her pulse!" He put his fingers on Monir's wrist. After a moment passed, he said, "All right. She has a pulse, too!"

Robin took a deep breath, a sigh of relief. Then he said, "She bled from her head!"

"It seems like she took a fall and cracked her head. But, how did this happen?" the officer commented with a question.

"I don't know!" Robin answered.

"Before you came, I searched around the house, but there was no sign of a breaking in. Something must have happened to cause her to fall. Maybe she slipped!"

"Maybe!"

"Well, I'd better bring my first-aid medical box and the oxygen from the car. I'll make a call also to arrange her transport to a hospital."

"Thank you, officer."

After the officer left the kitchen, Robin grabbed a towel and dampened it with water. He applied it to his mother's forehead. He called Monir's name several times as he patted her face. But no luck! Monir did not regain consciousness.

The officer walked into the kitchen carrying his first-aid box. "Did she wake up?" he asked.

"Not yet."

"Well, maybe the oxygen would help her," the officer said as he put the oxygen mask on her face.

"Did you call the ambulance?" Robin asked.

"I sure did. The ambulance will be here any moment," the officer said. Then, he continued, "Do you have any idea how long she's been unconscious?"

"My bet is about an hour and a half."

"Wahh! That much? It sure must have been hard for your son to be without any supervision throughout the whole time! You are lucky that he is OK!"

"I wish she would be OK, too."

Monir gradually opened her eyes. A smile appeared on Robin's face.

"You see. Never lose your hope!" the officer commented. "She is coming back!"

"Mom, are you OK?" Robin asked.

"...Ah...ah...hhh! What happened?" Monir asked.

"You probably had a fall. But, that's OK! Just relax!"

In less than an hour Monir was in the hospital. By the time she was taken to the emergency room, she was fully awake. The emergency room physician in charge called me in my office after he had evaluated her. He tried to explain what had happened to Monir.

"Dr. Tabib, a patient of yours was brought to the ER due to a syncope episode. Her name is Mrs. Abramov. She apparently fell. She has a big cut on her head, which I already sutured. As far as I understand, she was unconscious for about an hour and a half. She lost the control of her urine with the fall. I think she had some kind of seizure!"

"Are you sure you are talking about Mrs. Abramov?" I asked skeptically, surprised about what I was hearing.

"Yes! That's her!"

"I saw her just two days ago in my office. I found her generally in good shape. I cannot believe she had a seizure!"

"I don't know either. Maybe she had a stroke, although she moves her arms and legs. It could be that or something else as well!"

"A stroke? How can it be? Her blood pressure was under control! She does not have any other risk factors for a stroke! Unless…unless she bled into her brain. Did you get a CT of her head?"

"She is on her way to have it done. By the way, are you planning on coming in to see her?" he inquired.

"Of course!" I answered. "I'll be there as soon as possible. By then, she would have done the CAT scan, too."

"Good enough! I'll see you later."

As I hung up, I recalled that Monir was so afraid of getting a stroke. Now, she was in the hospital because of a major medical problem with an unclear nature. "Did she really have a stroke?" I asked myself.

Decision! Decision! Decision! Apparently, it did not make any difference what I decided. I used medicine to lower Monir's blood pressure. I utilized the art of medicine to lower her anxiety. But, neither of these methods changed her destiny. It is all about the patients' fate in the game of superiority between destiny and a physician. In Monir's case, I could hear destiny's raucous laughter with its deceitful move.

As I entered the emergency room later that evening, I saw Robin and Jasmine standing next to Monir's bed. Robin was very anxious. He was literally in tears. Both of them had many questions to ask. I tried my best to answer them one by one. The main question remained as to why Monir had a seizure! After I reviewed her chart, I asked them to step outside of the room for a talk. Robin immediately began questioning me, "Did you look at the CT of her head?"

"Yes, I did," I answered.

"Do you have any idea why she lost consciousness?" Robin asked.

"Yes! Unfortunately, there is a problem within her brain," I replied.

"A problem? What kind of problem? Did she have a stroke?" Jasmine asked.

"No! She did not have a stroke. But, I don't have good news to give you! I still don't have the official report from the radiologist regarding the CT."

"So, what do you think it is?" Jasmine asked.

"Unfortunately, it seems she has a brain tumor!" I answered.

"A brain tumor!" Robin said with shock. "How can it be? She has never had any problem, not even a simple headache! Isn't it true that tumors may come with headaches?" he asked.

"That's right; but only in some cases. I'm telling you what I know so far!"

"How big is this tumor?" Robin asked.

"Almost as big as an apple!" I answered.

"An apple! Wahh!" Jasmine said. "That is large! Such a big tumor! We did not even have any knowledge of it! So, doctor, what are you going to do about it now?"

"I'll ask a Neurosurgeon to come in to evaluate her."

"Is this brain tumor dangerous? Is she going to live? Do you think she needs surgery?" Robin asked several questions in a row.

"I know you have many unanswered questions now. But, the best thing is to do as much as possible to help her," I said as I tried to avoid predicting Monir's future.

"OK! But, doctor, please do not tell my mom anything! She is so scared!" Robin requested.

"I know. She is afraid to be disabled!" I responded.

"Tell her that she has some kind of piece of fat in her head. Just tell her something that does not make her frightened," Robin said.

I felt that I not only had to care for Monir, but I needed to comfort Robin as well with my medical management. Therefore, knowing Monir's emotional state, I agreed with Robin's plans not to alarm her. However, I never told her that she had a "piece of fat" in her head!

It was a little before midnight when I left the emergency room. On my way home, I quarreled with myself about how there could have been no prior indications of such a big brain tumor. "How can you give a clean bill of health to someone, and two days later, she collapses with seizures?" I asked myself resentfully. "But, Monir did not have any symptoms to make me aware that something was going on. How could I have possibly known that she had such a problem?" I argued with myself. I considered that there had to be more facts involved in this scenario!

The next day, I visited Monir in the hospital. She was sitting on the bed having her breakfast. Robin was at her bedside, too. She stopped eating as soon as she saw me.

"Doctor, what happened to me? Why do I have to be here? Am I going to die? Another doctor came in and said that I needed surgery for my head. Please, help me, doctor! Please!" she said. Then, tears filled her eyes and cascaded down her cheeks.

"Take it easy Mrs. Abramov. It will be OK. If you need an operation, it is for your benefit," I said.

"Doctor, just do something for me to stay alive, please!" she pleaded as she was crying.

After I examined Monir, Robin and I left the room.

"The neurosurgeon was here earlier this morning," Robin said.

"Yes, I read his notes already."

"So, what do you think?"

"Things look better than I expected. It appears she has a benign tumor!"

"The neurosurgeon's impression was the same. This means it is not a bad one! Is that right?"

"Yes. However, she still needs to go for the surgery."

"Are you sure about this? You know, doctor, the nurses and the medical residents also recommended the same surgeon you called in to see her. But, don't you think we'd better discuss this with another neurosurgeon before making any final decision? Maybe she does not need a surgery."

"Robin, please understand! She has a brain tumor. It has to be removed. A tumor may grow without a surgical intervention. The result of the CT scan is clear. I do not recommend that you find excuses for a different approach," I said firmly. I spoke decisively to Robin partly due to my frustration and partly out of fear for Monir's fate if she did not have surgery.

"Alright! I was kind of hesitant to send my mother for a brain surgery. I hope you understand?"

"I understand. I'm worried about her, too. But, under these circumstances, the best choice is to remove the tumor!"

"OK. Doctor Tabib! Whatever you decide. Just don't make her frightened, please! She will be freaked out. Tell her that we have to remove the fat in her head."

"I'll do my best!"

◆   ◆   ◆

I learned more about Monir's condition over the following days after her hospitalization. I discovered that her brain tumor had not developed over the last year or two, but throughout many years and probably decades. She was suffering from a slow growing tumor, called meningioma. It commonly lacks any clinical presentation, which makes it tricky, if not impossible to identify. In some cases, this tumor is found accidentally, only after death! If any medical problem arises as a result of this tumor, it usually appears in the fifth or sixth decade of life. This is what occurred in Monir's case. Up until the time I learned these facts, my conscience was in turbulence because of the possibility of misjudgment on my part. However, It was comforting to know that some medical conditions are difficult to diagnose, even with the best intentions of a physician. Some circumstances just play "hide and seek"! I wondered if the costly method of total body scans might be the answer to finding some of these silent medical problems, as in Monir's case! However, does this technique not provide us with "the picture of the moment"? No one can know or predict what might happen to oneself in a few years down the road!

Meningioma can be positioned in different regions of the brain. Monir was fortunate to have an easily dissectible tumor because of its convenient location in her skull. Her recovery after the surgery was fast and without any complications. One day after her operation, I saw her in her hospital bed. Her head was covered with dressing. She pointed to her head and said in a heartbreaking voice, "Dr. Tabib, do you see what the surgeon did to me? I hope he did a good job! He finally removed the piece of fat from my head!"

A few days later, Monir was discharged home. She still needed to be followed for her general condition and the recent seizure activity prior to her fall. Therefore, she continued her follow-up visits with me. She remained on anti-seizure medications. Her blood pressure, cholesterol, and asthma all remained under control. After her recovery she felt confident about her future. During her visits, she gave me the impression that she was looking forward to seeing her grandchildren, especially Jonathan, growing.

MEDICAL WISDOM

There is a constant normal electrical wave in the brain. During a phenomenon, called **seizure**, a group of the cells in the brain fire an abnormal autonomous electrical discharge. This discharge may spread to the whole brain or to localized areas of the brain. Based on the severity or the type, the seizure is associated with mild, moderate, or severe convulsions of one or more parts of the body. A person may or may not lose consciousness during the incident. The unconscious episode may result in a fall, thus causing an injury. Loss of urine or feces may occur as well. A single non-febrile seizure may happen to as many as 5–10% of the population during their lifetime. This mostly occurs in childhood or late adulthood[8], [12].

Causes—Some seizures have reasons and some are without any identifiable causes. Inflammation of the brain itself (encephalitis), inflammation of its covering layer (meningitis), and quick shifts of the electrolytes in the blood are a few of the reasons for convulsions. An acute change in the body's temperature, for example, as in the rapid development of fever due to a sickness, especially in children, may cause febrile seizure. Change in the structure of the brain tissue, such as a tumor, a vascular malformation, a stroke, or some degenerative diseases of the brain (e.g., Alzheimer's disease) are the other etiologies of seizure formation. A person with *recurrent* seizure activities may be considered to have **epilepsy**.

Types—Seizures are called *partial* if they occur within discrete regions, and *generalized* when they arise from both sides of the brain simultaneously[8]. Absence and grand mal seizures are examples of the last category. The followings are some examples of these types:

A forty-year-old Oriental woman, who was a cashier in the pharmacy, was transferred from her work place to the emergency room because she could not control her hand. When I saw her in the hospital, she said that she had had a few similar episodes in the past six months. Her hand twisted upward and her arm folded toward her body involuntarily with each episode. Her last experience was brief, but sure enough to make her frightened. Except once, during these episodes, she usually never lost consciousness. She also mentioned that she suffered from meningitis in her childhood. Her electroencephalogram (EEG) was consistent with abnormal waves coming from one region of the brain. This can be an example of a *partial* seizure. Carbamazepine, valproic acid and phenytoin are usually used for the treatment of this kind of seizure.

One morning, the mother of a nine-year-old patient of mine took him to school. After he entered the school, he fell. During this episode, he lost consciousness, his eyes rolled up, and his body shook for a few seconds. An hour later, after he had been taken to the emergency room, I spoke to his mother. She said that her child had not eaten much that morning. First, we thought low blood sugar had caused him to faint. However, more thorough investigation over the following days, which included an EEG, showed that he was suffering from an *absence* seizure. This kind of seizure often presents itself without generalized convulsions, unlike the situation for the child. Absence seizures are characterized by interruption of an activity, staring, and unresponsiveness lasting a few seconds, but without loss of muscle tone. This type of epilepsy usually has a favorable prognosis. It may cease spontaneously before the age of 20 years for the ones without convulsions. The treatment is frequently valproic acid.

Grand mal seizures are generalized convulsions with loss of consciousness. They are usually associated with motor activity. This kind of seizure is similar to receiving an electric shock. Therefore, as a result of electrical stimulation, the muscles of the patient become spastic (tonic phase). The attack is associated with the bowing of the body forward and bending of the head and the heels backward (opisthotonus) and the halting of breathing. As a result, the patient turns a bluish color because of the lack of oxygenation to the tissues. Due to the muscle contraction, including the muscles of the jaw, the tongue may be bitten. The next phase is a series of jerking motions (clonic phase). The loss of urine or feces may be noticeable during this phase. The entire process may last a few minutes. Some diseases of the brain, as stated earlier, may cause similar presentation as in grand mal convulsions. This was possibly the type of seizure that was triggered by the meningioma in Monir's case, leading her to lose consciousness!

Most patients with generalized convulsive disorders may be controlled with only one agent, such as phenytoin. However, valproic acid, lamotrigine, carbamazepine, or phenobarbital may be used as alternative treatments either alone or in combination with one another. A close follow up by a physician is required after initiation of such treatments.

Prevention—Little is known about how to prevent a seizure. However, stress, sleep deprivation, toxic materials, such as alcohol or drugs, may precipitate seizure activity, especially in susceptible individuals. Prevention of a rapid rise of temperature in children is recommended to prevent any possible development of a febrile seizure.

11

Alcohol

The den was a fairly large room. A landscape painting was hung on its wall. A portrait of a man was on the shelf. The feverish voice of a TV sport reporter filled the air, "…This is a kind of game that you rarely see. It was impossible to save that ball and score a point, but he did…" Walter, a forty-year old, very tall, slender bespectacled man was sitting on a long sofa located in the corner of the room. He was watching an evening game. His feet were propped up on the coffee table. A glass of vodka was in his hand. A half empty bottle of liquor was on the table. Two empty beer cans also stood next to the bottle. As Walter finished his drink, he roared excitedly, "Yes! That is a good point." No one else was in the room to hear him! Then, he poured the remainder of the vodka into his glass.

Walter's wife, Nikkei, was preparing dinner in the kitchen. She entered the den and said with frustration, "Are you still drinking? When are you gonna stop?" Then, she picked up the empty bottle and continued, "I really don't know what to do with you! You are a mess!"

Walter raised his right hand and pointed to the TV. "Look at this player in action! I love this game!" he said excitedly as if he did not hear his wife. "Hey! Nikkei! Don't you think this is a great game?"

"A great game? Your life is made up of games, alcohol, and delivering letters! That's all! There is nothing else important to you in this world. Now, if you're hungry you can join me so we can have dinner together." Then, she carried the empty bottle and cans into the kitchen.

As she was walking away, Walter said, "I'm not hungry. I want to watch the game!"

"Yeh! You're never hungry. Never!"

◆   ◆   ◆

Walter worked as a mail carrier in the local post office. The next day, he was very excited to get to work so he could talk about last night's game with his friends. When he arrived, he saw his friend, Frank, who already was in full gear, working on some boxes.

"Hey, Frankie! Did you see last night's game?" asked Walter.

"Of course I did! Who is gonna miss such a great game? The last point was just amazing! Only the good players can throw the ball like that!" Frank said.

"I just loved it. Nothing makes me happier than to watch a good game and drink some vodka!"

"The doctors say that drinking moderately is good! Isn't that so?" asked Frank.

"Sure they did!" Walter said.

Frank bent over to pick up a heavy load. "Look! Would you come over here and give me a hand moving this box? It's kind of heavy!"

"Of course! Let me put these envelopes aside," said Walter as he put a few envelopes on the counter. "…And, I'll be there to help you. All right! I'm coming!" As he walked around to the other side of the counter, Walter suddenly became motionless. He stopped, closed his eyes, and began falling to the floor. As he collapsed, he hit his face very hard on the corner of the counter. The force of impact knocked off his eyeglasses. He landed on the floor face up. Unexpectedly, Walter's eyes rolled up and he stopped breathing. Frank was watching him. The breath was trapped in Frank's chest and he could not talk. He took a step toward Walter and bent over to look at him. Walter was not breathing. Frank began shaking him and called his name, "Walter! Walter! Wake up!" But, he did not know what else to do. Finally, he began yelling for help.

"Help! Help! Somebody, help!" Frank shouted loudly.

Nancy and Peter, two coworkers, ran into the room.

"What's wrong with you? Why are you yelling?" Nancy asked immediately as she entered the room. Then she noticed Walter on the floor. "Oh, my goodness! What happened to Walter?"

"Look, he's shaking! He can't breathe!" Peter yelled.

Walter kept shaking. Nancy bent over and came closer to Walter. Then, she said, "He's having a seizure! We'd better call 911."

"I'll do it," Peter said.

In a few minutes two medics entered the post office. Along with them, they rolled in a narrow stretcher. A portable oxygen tank and a medical box were on the stretcher. When they saw Walter on the floor, they immediately prepared the mask to give him oxygen. Once they knew the story, one of the medics opened his medical box and pulled out an ammonia inhalant capsule. He broke it apart, removed the oxygen mask, and brought it close to Walter's nose. As he inhaled the ammonia, Walter gradually regained consciousness. Once he became stable, they placed him on the stretcher and carried him to an ambulance.

"Sir," pointed Frank to one of the medics. "Take his eyeglasses before you leave, please. He cannot see without glasses."

"Wow!" the medic commented. "How can he see with these glasses? One of the lenses is completely cracked!"

"Well! It's better than nothing!" Frank answered.

In less than an hour, Walter was lying on a stretcher in the emergency room. His face was aching, but he had no recollection of what just happened to him. Later, the emergency room physician evaluated him and found a cut on Walter's forehead. It was large enough to require suturing.

As part of my hospital on-call duties, I was responsible for the admission of patients to the hospital that day. When I received the telephone call from the emergency room physician, he told me about Walter.

"Dr. Tabib! You are the doctor on-call for medicine today!" he said.

"You got that right. How can I help you?"

"Listen! There is a gentleman here who does not have a doctor. He fainted in the post office today. Apparently he works there. It seems he is a drinker. I got a story that he had some shakes after his fall, similar to a seizure. This could be related to alcohol abstinence," he explained.

"How is he doing now?"

"He's alert. He does not remember what happened to him. I think he should be admitted to the hospital for evaluation."

"Is he stable?"

"Yes. Absolutely."

As a norm in the admission of stable patients to the hospital, I asked the resident on-call to evaluate Walter before I arrived at the hospital.

"OK! I'll take care of him," I responded favorably. "I also like to discuss the case later with the resident."

"No problem. I'll call the resident for you."

"Thank you. I'll be there later today."

Throughout my many years of practice, I have come to learn the information reported by the emergency room physician might be just the tip of an iceberg concerning a patient's medical history. So it was in Walter's case!

Throughout the day, I followed Walter's condition by discussing the case over the phone with the admitting resident. Later in the evening, after a long day of work, I went to visit Walter in the hospital. Once I verified which unit he was in, I went to the appropriate nursing station. As is my routine, I pulled out his chart for review. I could not find any new information beyond what was gathered in the resident's report. It appeared Walter's facial contusion was the only significant physical finding!

I walked along the quiet hospital hallway until I reached Walter's room. The room was dark with only the hallway light illuminating it. I found Walter resting on his side on the bed. I placed my hand very gently on his leg. His reaction was a quick turn of his head toward me. Even in the darkness of the room, I could discern a hazy discolored area around his right eye. After I apologized for waking him, I introduced myself as his physician in charge. To keep his peace of mind, I did not ask him to turn on the light.

"Doctor! I wasn't asleep. I just had my eyes closed."

"Well, I hope that I did not disturb you! I have a few questions to ask."

"OK."

"Do you know what happened to you?"

"They said that I fell!"

"Is that all? Is this what you were told or do you remember falling?"

His answer was not straightforward. "I hit my face to the counter, too!"

"It is late now and I'm sure that you want to rest! So, I'll get to the point. I received some information that you might have been drinking. Would you give me some information about your drinking habit!"

"Oh, doctor! I don't drink much."

"Would you tell me how much alcoholic beverages you might consume?"

"It is probably one or two glasses a week."

"Anything else?"

"Maybe a beer on the weekends, too!"

During the entire conversation, I did not detect much emotion in Walter's face. His answers were brief and succinct. I did not feel comfortable asking him any more questions. I thought I possibly would irritate him. I proceeded with the physical exam. As I was examining his abdomen, suddenly, I was shocked to palpate a very large liver. This finding had not been picked up, prior to my examination, since his admission to the hospital. One thing came to my mind immediately; "He must drink very heavily and thus caused damage to his liver!"

"Have you been aware of any problem with your liver?" I asked.

"Not that I know of! Did you find anything wrong, doctor?"

"Well! Your liver appears enlarged."

"What does it mean?"

"It would be better to evaluate you with a test. Then, I'll have an answer for you."

"What kind of a test is it?"

"An ultrasound would be a reasonable test to begin with."

"OK!"

"I'll try to arrange it for you tomorrow!"

I terminated my explanation prematurely. I needed to obtain more information about his liver. I left the room after answering a few more of Walter's questions. I left him with the uncertain knowledge of having "an enlarged liver".

Walter tossed and turned in his bed for an hour, thinking about his new problem. He was wondering how serious it could be when the liver grows in size. Before he fell asleep, he anxiously asked himself, "Is this going to cut my life short?"

The next day, as soon as I entered Walter's room, he swiftly sat down on his bed. He appeared more alert compared to the night before. The black and blue marks of the trauma to his face had extended to his forehead and partially to his left eye.

"Well! Doctor! What is your plan for me?" he asked.

"I have to study more about the reason behind the shakes that you had. I already asked a neurologist to see you. I'm also interested in finding out more about the condition of your liver. You will have an ultrasound of your abdomen today."

"I know that the liver is very important. Do you think something is wrong with my liver?"

"All I can tell you now is that it's enlarged. Tomorrow, we will have a better answer," I replied.

More shocking news came the next day after I had spoken to Walter's wife.

"Doctor! My name is Nikkei. I'm Walter's wife. I understand you are taking care of him in the hospital," she said when she contacted me by phone.

"That is right, ma'am."

"How did you find my husband?"

"Apparently, he had some kind of seizure activity. He is supposed to have an electroencephalogram tomorrow to find out its cause."

"Do you think this has anything to do with the amount of liquor that he drinks?"

"Liquor! I'm glad that you brought up the subject. Would you tell me more about the amount of alcohol he consumes?"

Her answer was like the bursting of water through a dam! "Oh! Doctor! He drinks! He drinks, doctor! He may easily finish a bottle of vodka in one evening. I cannot stop him! I don't know what to do with him!"

"So, his situation is bad!" I commented.

"Doctor, bad is not the word to describe him! His condition is dreadful! He drives me crazy. He makes me sick to my stomach with his behavior. Sometimes, I really don't know what to do with him," she said with aggravation. Then, she continued. "Regarding the seizures! You should know he has already had two other episodes. Once he had a seizure right in front of me during our meal. I was afraid that he would choke. The second time, was when he was asleep. He wet himself, also. I asked him to see a doctor, but he refused! He is a tough case! I don't know what else to do with him!"

"So, you're telling me he had at least two previous episodes of seizures!" I asked to confirm the facts.

"That's quite right."

"Well! Ma'am! This is an important piece of information that you have given me."

"Doctor, what is the story regarding his liver? He tells me that his liver got big."

"The issue is under work-up evaluation. However, I truly believe that his liver has been affected by drinking alcohol over the years. I've already requested an ultrasound test to clarify the nature of the problem."

"Doctor, I'm sorry to take so much of your time. I appreciate that you're speaking to me."

"The pleasure was all mine, ma'am. You've really given me good insight about your husband. I want to assure you that I'll give Walter the proper care."

Drinking alcoholic beverages on a continuous basis is an addictive behavior. That is probably the end-point of some kind of psychological pressure in life, such as depression, although certain predisposing genetic factors may also contribute to this kind of demeanor. The stressful event may have passed a long time ago. However, the consumption of alcohol may be incorporated into the daily routine of a patient with dependence. Alcoholics may not even remember what initiated their addiction. The fact is, in many instances, excessive drinking is a sign of crying out for help. Unfortunately, many of the patients who depend on alcohol to pass their day, have often caused damage to their body systems by the time of diagnosis. This was the case with Walter. His long-term addiction resulted in the enlargement of his liver and probably triggered convulsions. Heavy drinking of alcohol may cause harm not only to the liver, but also to some other organs, such as the heart and the blood vessels.

On the third day of Walter's hospitalization, I did not find him in his room! When I asked the nurses where he was, the answer was not surprising. He actually was in the right place! He was attending an in-hospital meeting with the "alcohol services unit". He was encouraged by the counselor to receive therapy in order to remain alcohol free. Surely, this was a new challenge for Walter. He would have to deal with his long-term unfavorable behavior. As I was writing a note in his chart, the meeting concluded. Walter came over to the nursing station. He approached me and asked a question, "Doctor, did you receive the report of my ultrasound?"

I looked at him. I was glad that he was interested in his condition. "Yes, I did. I think we should hold this discussion in your room," I answered.

"So, do you want me to wait in my room?"

"That's right. I'll see you in a minute!"

When I entered Walter's room a few minutes later, he was sitting at the edge of his bed. Once he saw me, he asked me impatiently, "Well, how bad is the news?"

"It depends upon how you look at it."

"What ever it is, I have to deal with it."

"Unfortunately, your liver has been damaged, probably as a result of your heavy consumption of alcohol throughout the years. The normal tissue of the liver has a soft texture. In your case, this tissue has been changed to one which is rough and has bands. This is a condition called "fibrosis". The cells of your liver have also filled with fat, transforming it into a "fatty liver.""

"That sounds pretty awful!"

"For now, your liver is larger than normal. This indicates severe consequences associated with serious malfunction. However, as I said earlier, it depends upon how you look at the picture!" I said with a smile.

"You mean there is a good side, too?"

"The good part is, in your case, if you can stop drinking, you'll be able to reverse the deterioration of your liver to some extent. And then, it will shrink."

"That sounds better!"

Once he finished his last comment, he paused. He turned his head, looked away, and then said very firmly, "I think I learned my lesson the hard way! I know the liver is a very important organ in my body. I am not stupid! Enough is enough! Alcohol will be history in my life. I mean it!"

Walter was not discharged without treatment for his seizures. As I unfolded the story of the previous convulsions that Walter experienced at home, the neurologist did not wait to receive the report of the electroencephalogram. He immediately initiated treatment for possible grand mal seizures, since it seemed that alcohol triggered their manifestations.

Walter, at the age of forty, continued to watch his favorite sport games on TV. As usual, he sat in front of the TV set and enjoyed watching the players in the games. This time, however, there was a big difference. He kept a glass of water or soda instead of alcohol in his hand. In the other hand, he had his anti-seizure medication! Walter was lucky. Unlike some cases, his liver condition was reversible. However, he learned not to take chances with his life and his health!

MEDICAL WISDOM

A small amount of alcohol, especially red wine, may not be harmful. In fact, it may even be beneficial and healthful. However, the heavy drinking of alcoholic beverages, especially the ones with a high concentration of alcohol may certainly have ominous consequences.

Alcohol is a beverage with a high source of calories, but it lacks the important nutrients, such as proteins or vitamins. In other words, a heavy drinker may substitute the energy from alcohol but ends in dietary deficiency. This leads to serious health problems including, but not limited to, immune deficiencies, heart failure, brain dysfunction, liver damage, and muscle weakness. A healthy body needs wholesome nourishment. Therefore, an alcoholic has to stop drinking for the sake of his life. To make a long story short, should an alcoholic continue to drink, the life span is shortened by an average of 15 years, with the leading causes of death, in decreasing order, being heart disease, cancer, accidents, and suicide[8].

One of the devastating complications of chronic abuse of alcohol is the damage to the liver and eventually the possibility of liver failure. These consequences are divided into 3 forms. The first one is **alcoholic fatty liver**, which is a reversible condition. In this case the liver become full of fat. The second form is **alcoholic hepatitis**, in which the liver gets so sick that some of the liver cells die. As the body tries to cope with the situation, it sends many white blood cells, as part of the immune system, to help the damaged liver. However, as the person continues drinking alcohol, the third form of liver damage, known as **cirrhosis**, evolves. In this case an enormous number of liver cells are destroyed, because of alcohol! The liver shrinks and becomes firm due to the deposition of hard fibrotic bands. Based on the alcoholic's behavior, a combination of the spectrum of these damages can be seen. This was the condition in Walter's case because he had varying degrees of liver disease.

As I stated, alcohol is a form of "junk drink". It may have deleterious effects on many organs of the body. In the gastrointestinal system, it destroys the internal lining of the stomach and the gut causing bleeding. It may also cause chronic inflammation of the pancreas, called pancreatitis. In the blood, the shape, the structure, and the function of different cells are altered as an outcome of heavy alcohol ingestion, resulting in decreased immunity. An alcoholic may end up with multiple broken bones as a result of recurrent falls.

One of my young patients fell on the stairway of his basement after heavy drinking. He was missing for many hours, until his father found him unconscious in the basement. The next day he was brought to my office for evaluation. After a thorough examination, my final comment was "Go to the emergency room!" It was not surprising that the computerized tomography (CT scan) of his head showed a broken skull and a cerebral hemorrhage (bleeding in the brain tissue). A full neurological evaluation led to the initiation of an anti-convulsive remedy! Two years later, to prevent the possibility of new seizure activity, he was still under treatment with the same medication that he began earlier.

There is some good news, too. Most of the undesirable changes in the body systems from chronic use of alcohol are partially or completely reversible if the patient avoids drinking completely.

Short-term use of benzodiazepines, such as diazepam (Valium®), chlordiazepoxide (Librium®), or oxazepam (Serax®), is an effective treatment modality to avoid the symptoms of alcohol withdrawal. This kind of drug is started at the same time as the treatment is initiated to bring an end to the drinking behavior. These medications and others are also used to treat **delirium tremens**, which is the state of confusion associated with severe withdrawal symptoms. Alcoholics are depleted in vitamins. Therefore, the patients have to take vitamins, especially thiamine and folic acid. For those patients in recovery, emotional support and close follow-up for an extended period of time, plays an essential role in maintaining the abstinence from alcohol.

Does someone really need all of the complications resulting from heavy and chronic consumption of alcohol? You are advised to seek medical attention if you fall into the following categories:

1.   You are a person who is dependent on alcohol to start your day.

2.   You feel guilty about your drinking.

3.   You have been annoyed by other's criticism about your drinking behavior.

4.   You tried unsuccessfully to cut down on the usage of alcohol.

A good source of information is to call your physician or call your nearest hospital. The names of some supportive organizations are listed at the end of this book. A helpful hand is waiting for you. Do not wait until it is too late!

12

A Christmas Gift

"Surrender!" A police officer shouted into the bullhorn. "You'd better come out! Raise your hands and give up!"

The time was 12:00 midnight. The two men were trapped after an unsuccessful attempted robbery of a pharmacy. Long before they could make their escape, the pharmacy's silent alarm had summoned a squad of police cars to the area. A bright beam of light from a helicopter hovering above the street was focused on the pharmacy, making every object visible in the darkness. Marshall and Peter were hiding behind the counter of the pharmacy. Marshall was a tall strapping man. His blue eyes were scanning around the store. His long shoulder-length blond hair flicked with each of his jerky moves. Peter was slightly shorter. He immersed his left fingers into his dark black hair. Then, his hazel eyes gazed at the tall large glass front window, which was brightened by the light beam. They had broken into the pharmacy looking for money and morphine.

"Come out!" the police officer yelled. The frustration was clear in his voice. "You'll never see the sunlight again if you stay there! You'll be caught, dead or alive!"

Inside the pharmacy, Marshall could feel his heart pounding. His face was covered with sweat. Peter was flushed and the white sclera of his eyes was blood shot. He held a small pistol in his right hand. While he was in a squatting position, he began moving from side to side. Then, he said, "I gotta go to the bathroom! I'm gonna wet myself!"

Marshall, who was next to him, turned toward Peter, and said through clenched teeth, "Do you see this? That's all your fault! You haven't been thinking enough!" He pulled a bunch of cash from his pocket and shoved it toward Peter. Anger was in his eyes. "Look at this money! We came all the way here for this money and you want to go to bathroom! Couldn't you do it earlier?"

"These cops made me nervous!" Peter said with frustration. "What do you want me to do?"

"You are crazy!" Marshall yelled, "Just a crazy man! And, I followed you!"

"You know what! Give me the morphine before I pee in my pants!"

"Now?" Marshall said with vehemence, "Are you a fool? The cops are outside. And you want to shoot up, now?"

"Hey! Listen! We're gonna get caught! I'd better use it before they take it away from me!"

"This is your last chance!" the officer's voice echoed outside of the pharmacy. "We won't shoot you if you come out without a problem! Otherwise, your families will have to prepare for your funeral!"

"It doesn't sound like we can get out of this place in one piece! Damn it!" Marshall said. "I didn't think this would be the end of it after so much trouble. Here it is! Get the morphine and the syringe. Do whatever you want." Then he pulled a few small brownish colored vials and some syringes from his pocket. "Is this what you want?"

"I got to get one of these babies!" Peter put down the gun and picked up two vials. He broke their tips and put the needle of a syringe into the vials to suck up the contents. Then, he put the syringe between his teeth. He pulled up his sleeves with his free hand. As he exposed his arm, he grabbed the syringe. He pushed the needle into his skin and pumped the large quantity of liquid into his bulging vein.

"Come out! Not much time left for you!" the voice of police officer was heard again.

Peter became weak after the injection. He sat down and stretched out his legs while he leaned against the wall. He appeared very relaxed. He grabbed the gun from the floor and aimed at one of the large store windows. The headlights of the cars and the helicopter spotlight illuminated the window.

"What are you doing?" Marshall asked.

"Bang! Bang!" Peter said. "I'll kill them all!"

"We're already in trouble! Don't make it worse," Marshall growled.

Peter brought the gun down. He kept looking at the window. Then, suddenly he raised his hand. He aimed again at the window. His finger was on the trigger.

"No! Don't shoot! Don't shoot, Peter!" Marshall raised his voice.

"I'll kill them all! Every one of those bastards!" Peter aimed again and pulled the trigger. A blast was heard and the entire window was blown out, sending thousands of fragments of glass scattering onto the street and inside of the store. Immediately after, silence filled the store. Peter broke the silence by laughing hysterically. "Now, it is quiet. They are all dead! I told you I'd killed them all!"

"You fool! Look at yourself!" Marshall ridiculed, "You're a stinking mess. You've already peed in your pants!"

Peter laughed. His eyes were half closed. With a sluggish voice, he said, "I couldn't find the bathroom!"

Suddenly, the side-door of the pharmacy opened. A very furious voice was heard, "Freeze, or I'll shoot!" A police officer, with his gun aimed on the intruders, entered the pharmacy! Marshall stood up and raised his hands. Peter did not get up. His whole body was lying on the floor. Only his head was propped against the wall.

"Why are you standing, Marshall?" Peter said with a lethargic voice, indicating his intoxicated state. "This is only a ghost! I told you, they are all dead!"

"Don't move!" the police officer said.

"I'm not moving!" Marshall responded.

Three more police officers entered the store at once. They also aimed their guns toward Marshall and Peter. They were ready to shoot. Peter tried to raise his gun. "Well! If I have to kill ghosts, I'll do that!"

"No!" Marshall shouted as he raised his right leg and abruptly kicked Peter's fist. The pistol crashed a few feet away. "You made enough trouble!" Marshall said angrily.

"Good move!" one of the police officers said. "I'll point out what you did to the judge when we see you in the court! For now, get out of here!" Then, he put handcuffs on Marshall.

Both Marshall and Peter had histories of drug abuse and long criminal records. Six-month later, Marshall was sentenced to 7 years, while Peter received 15 years in prison. All this was due to the way of life that each had selected. They had to have known that addiction to drugs and attempted robbery would not have a better ending. They were lucky to stay alive or not be injured.

◆　　　◆　　　◆

Five years later

An evening, two weeks before Christmas, I was at home when my telephone rang. It was the emergency room physician at a local hospital notifying me of an admission.

"Doctor Tabib! Hi! This is Dr. Banner from the emergency room."

"Dr. Banner! Hi! How are you doing?"

"I'm fine." He cut the briefing short and continued, "I guess you know you're on call for medicine."

I knew time was precious to him. Thus, I answered him quickly, "Of course, I know I'm on call."

"Listen! There is a case for you. The woman doesn't have any primary physician. She is a 38 year-old-lady, alcoholic, and smoker, who was brought in with GI bleed! I think she has to be admitted."

"Is she stable?"

"Her hemoglobin was very low. She needed a transfusion of 2 packed of red blood cells."

"Well, I'd better come in!"

"OK! I think that's a good idea!"

"What is her name?"

"Olivia Jones."

An hour later, as I entered the emergency room, I looked for Olivia. I found her in the acute care section. I approached her. She was lying on a stretcher, covered by a hospital blanket. As I looked at her, I noted that she was a white woman. She was a Caucasian, round face and obese. A unit of blood was hung on a stand, transfusing the blood into her vein. She appeared very uncomfortable. She kept moving her head from side to side or bending it forward to look around, as if she had lost something! I introduced myself.

"Hi! My name is Dr. Tabib! Are you Miss Jones?"

"Yes, I am!" she said hastily as she looked at me with another quick move of her head!

"What happened to you?"

"I began passing black stools!"

"How long have you been experiencing this?"

"Quite a few days. Almost for two weeks!" she said. Olivia kept looking at me; her eyes wide open, indicating inner fears regarding what was happening to her. She continued being uneasy. Her speech was peppered with sharp, rapid verbal responses.

"They informed me you drink alcohol. Is that true?"

"Yes! That's true."

"How much do you drink?"

"Too much! Usually a few glasses a day! Sometimes a bottle or two!"

"That's quite a lot!"

"Yes, I know! I should quit!"

"Do you smoke, too?"

"About two packs a day!"

"You know the combination of alcohol and tobacco is not good! You'd better cut down!"

"I know! It will be changed!"

I paused and then I asked, "Who brought you in?"

"An ambulance!"

"With whom do you live?"

"My in-laws."

"So, you are married!"

"Yes, I am!"

"Where is your husband?"

"He's in jail!"

I grabbed her chart from the desk to review the notes. Then I asked her "In jail? Why is he in jail?"

"Because of a robbery! It's already been five years."

I shook my head and stopped asking any further questions. As I was looking at the notes in her chart, I discovered she was without any medical insurance. I felt sorry for her, but I had no other choices except to keep her in the hospital. "With the amount of alcohol she drinks, she needs treatment. She has been bleeding for several days! She has to be watched for this!" I thought to myself.

"Mrs. Jones, you have to stay in the hospital."

"OK. Whatever I have to do."

"You understand. You don't have any medical coverage!"

"Yes, I know!"

"So, who will pay for the expenses?"

"I don't know, yet."

"God, help you!" I said silently. I proceeded to examine her. Then, I sat down in the same room to write my notes. When I was ready to leave, I turned toward her and said, "Well, I'll see you tomorrow!"

"OK, doctor!" she said quickly.

Taking care of patients may provide moral and spiritual satisfaction for a physician. For me, taking care of Olivia was a "Good Samaritan" job.

The next day, when I went to visit Olivia, she was sitting at the bedside. Olivia already had received enough replacement for the blood that she lost. It was time for me to attend to another significant problem with her—a very high blood pressure!

"Hello, Doctor Tabibzadeh!" she said with a big smile on her face. "Did I say your name right?"

"Hey, you are one of the few people who said my name correctly!"

"So, listen! I feel great. When can I go home?"

"It looks like somebody is in a rush! I cannot discharge you yet! You are on protocol for alcohol rehab. It takes a few days before it is finished. Besides, your upper endoscopy, which was done a few hours ago, showed that you have an ulcer in the stomach. Luckily, it stopped bleeding. But, I don't know whether you will bleed again or not. It's too soon to go home."

"Are you telling me that you are keeping me here?"

"That's right!"

Olivia bowed her head. She appeared disappointed. Then she raised her head and said, "But I feel good!"

"Mrs. Jones, you have many problems. You drink! You smoke! And, you also have a very high blood pressure, probably because of alcohol! A blood pressure of 190/100 is very high and dangerous. I'm going to start you on blood pressure pills. You'd better take care of yourself. You cannot be born twice to this world. You have only one chance to live. You'd better grab it."

"I promise you, I'll quit drinking. I work hard. I have two jobs. I must go back to my work. I cannot afford to get fired."

"No one is holding you here by force. You can always sign a form called AMA. It means Against Medical Advise. Then, you are free to go."

"OK! OK! I'll stay. But, promise to discharge me as soon as possible."

"Fine! You got a deal, lady!"

As I finished my sentence, a big smile, indicating appreciation for my concerns, appeared on Olivia's face. It seemed that trust began to blossom in her heart. On my part, I was obligated by my moral duties, to bring her to a safe end.

An hour later, Olivia's telephone rang in the hospital room. It was her mother-in-law.

"How are you doing, Olivia?"

"Hi, Ma! Is that you?"

"Yah, it's me. I called to find out when you're coming home?"

"My doctor doesn't want to discharge me. He said I'm not well enough. He put me on special medications because of my alcohol problem. He also put me on blood pressure pills. He said that my blood pressure is high because of drinking alcohol. It looks like I have to stay here until I finish the course of medications for my rehab."

"You'd better stop drinking. You're staying in the hospital because of that."

"I promise not to touch any liquor any more. I promise! I even told this to the doctor. But, he didn't believe me!"

"Well! I wish that you'd keep your promise. I wish my son,…was…here to…help you."

"Ma! Don't cry, Ma! One day he'll join us. You'll see!"

"I…hope you're…right! He ruined his life because of drugs. I hope that, at least, you save yourself."

"Ma, from now on, things will change."

The next day, as Olivia saw me enter her room, she quickly changed her position to sit on the bedside. She began the conversation.

"OK! Are you sending me home today? Is that right?" she asked.

"Today! Do you want to go home? We haven't finished your rehab protocol yet. How can I possibly send you home? Once you're discharged, you'll go back to your routine. And, this means that you will drink and smoke. Then, you are back to square one, with more bleeding."

"I can't afford staying in the hospital!" she said as tears filled her eyes and started running down her cheeks. "I have two jobs that I have to keep. If I don't go back to my work tomorrow, they may fire me!"

"What? You want to go back to work tomorrow? I told you yesterday that you have an ulcer in your stomach. You have to take it easy for a while until it gets healed. You have to stop drinking. Also, the smoking doesn't help it—especially in your case, with a history of asthma. On top of everything, your blood pressure is too high."

"I promised to stop drinking. Didn't I?"

"I've heard a lot of similar promises from patients just like you. Those promises are only valid as long as the people are in the hospital!"

"No! That's not true about me. Please, just prescribe the medications and I'll take them at home."

"Are you sure about what you are saying?"

"I'm positive! I have to get home. I must go back to work to keep my job. I have no other way. Please, help me. I beg you!"

"Listen! Maybe you can go home. You stopped bleeding, but you need follow-up medical care. You need to take medications. I'm really worried about you."

"I will be a good girl. Believe me! I'll follow up with you."

Not knowing this woman prior to her hospitalization, I was troubled to discharge Olivia. I was faced with a dilemma. On one hand, she needed a healthy life style. On the other hand, she had financial pressure. How could I finalize her treatment in a short hospital stay and stabilize these two issues? How much could I trust an alcoholic patient to go home and not pick up a bottle of liquor? Could

I expect such a person to take her medications as I directed? How could I know she would follow through?

Olivia was already depressed because of her marital and family circumstances. For years, she sheltered herself behind alcohol as a way to escape from what had happened to her husband who was behind bars. She struggled to hold onto two jobs to maintain her dignity. If it were true, my keeping her in the hospital could cause her to lose her job, and thereby, become more destitute than she already was. Lack of enough monetary support might lead her to a more severe depressive state and very possibly escalate her drinking problem.

Discharging Olivia from the hospital was "my decision" of the day. It would have a significant effect on her destiny. It was a dilemma about which I needed to make a correct choice. This was not a hypothetical question, which might be asked in the medical board exam. It was a real life story! This was about Olivia Jones, a person among us with turbulent emotions who needed to be rescued. As I looked at her again, I saw tears running down her cheeks. My basic human instincts, finally, overcame my logical judgment. With a heavy heart and a pessimistic outlook, I felt I had to give her a chance! Could this be the only possibility for Olivia to find her right direction in life?

"OK, I had wanted to discharge you in 2 days. But, I'll discharge you today."

"Oh! Thank you! Thank You! You made my day. Believe me, I'll take the medications as you recommended."

"Some of these medications are expensive. Do you think you can afford them?"

"Whatever the price would be, I accept. I have to go back to work. I have two jobs. I may lose one of them if I don't attend. You don't know how important it is for me to leave today!"

"As I said, you take the medications every day. And, please do not touch alcohol. It would increase your blood pressure and you may bleed again!"

Suddenly she stood up, spread her arms and placed them around my shoulders and hugged me! "Dr. Tabibzadeh, you don't know how much I appreciate what you did for me!" she said in tears. It was indeed a great moment for her. I hugged her, too. Then I said, "Try to be a responsible person concerning yourself!"

◆   ◆   ◆

Five days later, and a few days before Christmas, Barbara, my secretary, who surprises me from time to time with her comments, approached me with a question.

"Listen! You saw a patient in the hospital a few days ago!"

"I see many patients in the hospital. Which one are you talking about?"

"Olivia Jones!"

"Olivia Jones? Oh! That patient? Poor lady! She is in trouble with many medical problems. OK! What about her?"

"She wants to see you."

"Are you kidding me? She has not seen a physician for years. Now, she wants to see me!"

"So! What do you want me to tell her?"

"I'm skeptical about this patient. I'm not sure she will follow my advice. Don't you think it will be a challenge to follow this patient?"

"Well, you're a master in challenges!"

"Am I? I want to see her healthy! But, I've my doubts if she has even taken any of her medications that I prescribed in the hospital."

"So, what are you saying?"

"All right, all right! Call her and tell her that if she wants to come in for a visit she has to follow through."

"Anything else?"

"That's it for now."

"I'll do it as you said!" Barbara said calmly as she walked toward her desk.

The next day, as I looked at my weekly schedule, I saw a familiar name on the list of Friday's patients, "Olivia Jones"! I turned toward Barbara and said, "So she eventually made an appointment!"

"Yes, she did. She really insisted upon seeing you. It seemed she wanted to prove something to you."

"Prove something? What does she want to prove?"

"You might be her only hope."

"Well, when I see her, I'll do my best. The question is will she do her best, too?"

Teaching medical students is also part of my practice. On Friday morning, I was busy talking with a young student in his mid-twenties in my consulting room. Barbara walked in and placed a new chart on my desk—"Olivia Jones".

"Is she here?" I asked.

"Believe it or not, she is here!" Barbara answered.

I could respond with nothing more than raised eyebrows.

"You look surprised!" the medical student commented.

"Surprised! I'm astonished!" I said. "She is a patient with a long history of alcoholism. This is probably her first time coming to see a doctor. These kinds of patients, unfortunately, may not continue with follow-ups. Olivia Jones is probably an exceptional patient regarding this matter!"

I called Olivia into the exam room. She gave me a big smile when she approached me. She wobbled as she walked because of her obesity. She was courteous enough to allow my medical student to remain in the room during her visit. She placed her medium-sized, brown handbag on the floor and sat down on the chair. She began the conversation with a remark as she kept a smile on the face, "I know. You don't have to tell me. You didn't believe I'd be here."

"That's right! It is a big surprise for me. Does this mean you followed my directions?"

"Yes, of course!"

"I gave you a few medications. Did you take any of them?"

"Every single one of them as you told me."

"And alcohol?"

"No way! I promised you. Didn't I? I threw away every bottle in the house. Nothing is left. My mother-in-law was so surprised."

"You mean that you have changed!"

"The bleeding from my stomach scared me. I almost died. You saved my life! You gave me a second chance to live normally. I'll never forget that!"

"OK, you are giving me very good news." Then, I said, while I directed her to sit on the exam table, "Now, let's proceed with checking your blood pressure today."

"It will be high because I'm nervous!"

The reading of Olivia's blood pressure was indeed high. "Your blood pressure is 180/100! You'd better lie down for a few minutes before I recheck you," I suggested. I turned the lights off as the medical student and I left the exam room. Olivia closed her eyes and tried to relax as much as possible. When we returned after a few minutes, I turned the lights on. I examined her and then I rechecked her blood pressure. I found it to be much lower.

"How much was it?" she asked.

"140/90!"

"Is this good?"

"That's the highest level of normal. I would like to see it even lower."

"I told you, I'm nervous. Are you going to change my medicines?"

"Not now! But, you try to stay calm as much as possible."

"Calm! That's against my nature! How can I be calm? My husband is in jail, I have to work in two places, and my mother-in-law is sick? Ask me something possible!"

"Olivia, you definitely have burdens. There is always a solution for any problem. You are a good person. Try to remain that way. Life can be changed if you behave differently. You would be surprised how people will react to you by your just being good. Maybe, even your boss will decide to give you a raise if you continue to do the right things."

"A raise!" she said and laughed loudly. "I wish! He'll never give us a raise!"

"How do you know? It's Christmas time. They say miracles happen during this time of the year."

"Well, I hope so!" she said as she shrugged her shoulders.

"To get on the right foot, I simply ask you to totally avoid drinking alcohol."

"That, I'll do."

Then, to wrap up the session, I said, "Do you know what? I'll start the first step for you. I'll give you a Christmas gift!"

"A Christmas gift? What could this be?" she questioned with a smile.

"As a courtesy, I don't want you to pay for your visit today! Take the money and do something good for yourself and your family. I'm ready to do that if this helps you in any way!"

"Wow! Thank you! That definitely helps. I appreciate it," she said with a laugh and immediately asked, "When do you want to see me again?"

"In a month! I'd prefer to see you frequently to be sure that no complications arise as a result of your medications. Besides, I'd like to monitor your behavior!"

"I'll be a good girl!"

When she left, I turned to the medical student and I asked, "What do you think?"

"That was a nice gesture not to receive any payment for her visit!"

"I know! I wanted to give her a sign to encourage her not to drink alcohol anymore! Unfortunately, she is an alcoholic," I said unhappily. "She needs a hand. Despite all the support that I try to give her, I'm skeptical about seeing her again!"

"That's sad."

"I believe that is the truth!" I replied.

Throughout the next few days, I continued thinking about Olivia's safety. She was the kind of person who, I thought, was at risk of returning to drinking alcohol at any moment. In spite of all my pessimistic feelings, to find a venue to reach out to her, I called Olivia on Christmas Eve. I wanted to remind her that I was interested in her well-being.

"Hello! This is Doctor Tabib! May I speak with Olivia, please?" I asked.

"Oh, Dr. Tabib! She has mentioned your name. Olivia? She is not home now. I'm her mother-in-law. Can I help you with anything?" asked the elderly woman on the other end of the telephone line.

"Where can I find her?"

"Olivia? She lives here! She'll come back in an hour."

"Would you tell her that I called to wish her Merry Christmas? Please, remind her to take her medications and avoid alcohol!"

"Oh, sure! She is doing very well! She takes her medications on time. I don't know what you told her, but she stopped drinking. I'll certainly tell her that you called."

"Thank you, and Merry Christmas," I said.

"Thank you, doctor," she said. "Happy holidays to you, too."

I expected a call back from Olivia to assure me about her behavior. I was disappointed when she did not call. The holidays passed without any sign of her. I knew that New Year's Eve could be another temptation for her alcoholic behavior. Nonetheless, I felt that calling her again might break the boundaries of her privacy.

Two weeks into the New Year, as I was losing my enthusiasm about Olivia's recovery, she surprised me again. She made her second appointment with me!

When I saw her in my office, I said, "You're back! I can't believe it!"

Olivia laughed and said, "I told you I would be back. You just never believed me!" Her anxious voice and the rapid pace of her speech had not changed.

"Well! I'm glad to see you here again…" I said. Her excitement about many things that had happened to her during the past weeks only allowed me to answer her with brief sentences.

"I know! I know you called me and spoke with my mother-in-law. She told me everything. That was very nice of you. I know you wanted to check on me. But, I was good! I didn't drink any alcohol at all since our last visit. Not even a sip. I feel great. I've never felt better in my life. Many good things have happened to me during the last month. They let my husband be with us for Christmas. We really had a great time together. But, he had to return to prison the next day."

"It's wonderful that you were together."

"As you said, good things would happen to me if I was good! Didn't you say that?"

"Yes, I did!"

"So, I've to tell you something very funny. I don't know how you knew this! My boss gave me a raise! Can you believe it? It was such a surprise that I really wanted to call you and let you know. But, I didn't want to bother you. I'm telling you, life is great!"

I smiled and then said, "So, things are working well for you."

"I'll tell you something else. My husband was put on the parole list! This is coming up in a few months."

"That's good, too! I don't recall if you ever mention his name to me."

"Marshall, Marshall Jones!"

"Why did he go to prison?"

"Robbery of a pharmacy. But, since that time he has changed a lot. Once, he was a drug addict. But, not anymore! He is clean now. He even goes to the church in jail. He has a great relation with his pastor. One day you'll see him. He is a tall man, muscular, and handsome."

Finally, I noticed a remarkable breakthrough in Olivia's life. I could recognize the pleasant aspect of the adventures that she experienced. Going to the hospital with a bleeding ulcer in her stomach had a tremendous effect on her. At the social level, she realized she had to change her attitude toward life. By using her willpower and strong mind to overcome her immature desires, she completely stopped drinking alcohol. She was on her way to conquering the beauty of her fate. She began going to Alcoholic Anonymous (AA) meetings on a regular basis. She kept in constant communication with her "sponsor" as well. On the medical part, her blood pressure came under control because she was taking her medications consistently. Her greatest desire for the future was to be with her husband under one roof.

◆   ◆   ◆

Seven months later

In July, for the fourth time since Marshall had been imprisoned, he was scheduled to appear before the parole committee for review. His last hope relied on the supportive letter that he had received from his pastor. One month after the evaluation, Marshall received a sealed envelope from the committee. He was fearful opening it. He did not want to read the same disappointing response he had experienced during the last six years. Before opening the envelope, he phoned Olivia from the prison.

"Did you get the letter?" Olivia asked.

"Yes, I did!" Marshall answered.

"So! You know how much we waited for this? What did it say?"

"I haven't opened it yet!"

"You what?"

"I said I haven't opened it yet!"

"Are you joking? My heart is pounding and about to jump out of my chest, and you still haven't opened the letter!"

"I wanted to open it with you!"

"Well! Come on! But, wait! I have to light a cigarette first!…OK! I'm ready now. Open it!"

Marshall began to slowly open the sealed letter. A few moments passed.

"I'm still waiting. But, I cannot wait too long! Because I'm gonna die from excitement!"

"Wait! Wait! I'm reading it…Olivia! Olivia! I'm gonna be free! They'll let me free. Do you understand this? I'm free."

"Hoo, Hoo! My husband is going to be free! That's the best news of the year! Do you know what I went through in the last few weeks for you? Finally, it happened."

"Six years! After six years I'm gonna be a free man again. A dream comes true."

"When are you gonna start packing your stuff?"

"They wrote in a month. Then, I will be home!"

◆   ◆   ◆

Some decisions made in life are proven to be correct only after some time. Looking back, it was a breakthrough decision to discharge Olivia from the hospital on time. Not only did she not lose her job, but also she found the right pathway in her life. She simply needed some encouragement. I am glad I could provide the support she required to succeed, even though I was very unenthusiastic and cynical about her image at times. Every person is different, however, he or she has to be given a second chance.

Marshall found a job right after his release from prison. Olivia continued her visits with me to regulate her blood pressure. They both attended AA meetings on a regular basis. They enjoyed the new friends they made in their group. One year after Olivia began attending those meetings, she was elected as the treasurer-secretary for the group. Marshall accepted the responsibility of organizing the reception arrangements. During Christmas of the following year, they had a big feast with their entire family. Most of Olivia's family was accustomed to the heavy drinking of liquor. Olivia passed her biggest test on that day. She did not touch alcohol at all! Marshall did not have to return to jail this time. He was a free man living with his wife.

Both Marshall and Olivia paid a heavy price for their detrimental behaviors. Marshall spent six years behind bars because of being a drug abuser. Olivia could have lost her life due to the bleeding from her stomach if there had not been medical intervention. Today, she still must struggle with high blood pressure as a consequence of long-term heavy drinking of alcohol, smoking cigarettes, and an inappropriate diet. Now, Olivia and Marshall are recovered from alcohol and drug use. They are both in high spirits viewing life from a different perspective. Olivia's next health challenge is to stop smoking!

MEDICAL WISDOM

"I feel good, Doctor!" This is the comment that I hear from the patients who suffer from systemic high blood pressure. Yet, eventually, they may feel the sensation of severe chest pain from a heart attack, a weakness of one side of their body as a result of a stroke, or shortness of breath because of congestive heart failure. These are some of the complications of long-term high blood pressure without appropriate treatment. The key is to postpone or eliminate those complications by aggressive medical management.

In order to measure blood pressure, an air bladder cuff is applied to the arm. An accurate reading is done when the cuff covers 2/3rd of the arm. A digital or aneroid blood pressure machine (sphygmomanometer) is used to measure the blood pressure. Blood pressure is measured in millimeters of mercury (mm Hg). Blood pressure reading has two numbers. The higher number is called systolic and the lower number is called diastolic. The blood pressure in children is lower than adults. It usually stabilizes after the age of 18 years. A normal blood pressure for adults is the systolic as high as 140 mm Hg, and the diastolic less than 90 mm Hg. An optimal blood pressure is 115/75 plus or minus 5 mmHg for patients with significant medical diseases, such as patients with diabetes, heart disease, or kidney disease. A consistent pressure with readings greater than those is called hypertension.

Hypertension, the disease of high blood pressure, develops due to the tightening and/or hardening of the arterial walls. Without finding a cause, it is called primary or essential hypertension. This form may represent more than 90% of the cases. In less than 10% of the population with high blood pressure, the cause may be other factors. A few of these include diseases of kidney tissue, tightening of the arteries of the kidneys (renal artery stenosis), elevation of the parathyroid hormone (hyperparathyroidism), or ingestion of oral contraceptives.

Hypertension, in combination with some other factors, may increase the chances of developing complications. Some of these factors include diseases, such as diabetes, hypercholesterolemia, and obesity, which have been discussed in the previous chapters. Others are genetic predispositions often found in the black race or in males. Having hypertension at a young age is an unfavorable prognostic factor. Both smoking and excessive alcohol intake adversely affect the blood pressure.

"Why do I have to take these pills?" This is a frequent complaint that physicians may hear from their patients. Hypertension damages many organs, called target organs. The heart, brain, kidneys, and eyes are the main organs, which are effected. A long-term hypertensive patient may have an enlarged heart, which may lead to a heart attack or congestive heart failure. Mini-strokes (transient ischemic attacks) and major strokes (cerebrovascular events) are other complications, which may lead to severe disabilities, such as memory impairment, loss of the function of a limb, partial blindness, or difficulty in speech. Deterioration in the function of the kidneys, as a result of untreated high blood pressure, may end up with dialysis. Vision may also be affected by hypertension due to the damage to the small arteries.

"Do I have to take these pills for the rest of my life?" The answer to this question is not clear-cut. It depends upon genetic factors and life style changes. Before initiating the use of any medication, behavioral modification should be the first line in treatment. Avoiding alcohol, ceasing smoking, adjusting one's diet to low cholesterol and low sugar foods, and exercising regularly may postpone medical treatment. Apparently, a low salt diet does not have a long-term significant effect on hypertension[15]. The following table is a guideline for a healthy *diet to reduce the blood pressure*[16]. The daily serving and the component of this diet have to be regulated for each individual and used in moderation.

Food group	Examples
Grains and grain products	Whole wheat bread, English muffin, pita bread, bagel, cereals, oatmeal
Vegetables	Tomatoes, potatoes, carrots, peas, squash, spinach, artichokes, beans, sweet potatoes
Fruits	Apricots, bananas, dates, grapes, oranges and its juice, grapefruit and its juice, mangos, melons, peaches, pineapples, prunes, raisins, strawberries, tangerines
Low-fat or nonfat dairy foods	Skim or 1% milk, low-fat yogurt, nonfat cheese
Meats, poultry and fish*	Non-fried lean meat, poultry, or fish
Nuts, seeds, and legumes	Almonds, filberts, peanuts, walnuts, sunflower seeds, kidney beans, lentils, mixed nuts

* Eating fish once per month or more can reduce the risk of ischemic stroke in men[17]

Medical treatment for hypertension

Since there are multiple factors in developing hypertension, there is no magic cure for it. However, many medications are used to regulate the uncontrolled elevated blood pressure. These remedies are aimed at reducing the damages of hypertension on the target organs. Patients educated about hypertension and its complications have a better chance of taking their medications on a regular basis.

There are different groups of medications for the treatment of hypertension. If not contraindicated, the best initial treatment is water pills (*diuretics*), since they may reduce the incidence of the complications from the heart disease[18]. These agents reduce the pressure by lowering the volume of the blood in the arteries. Patients may experience frequent urination upon beginning this treatment. Supplemental potassium and magnesium might be necessary in conjunction with various diuretics.

The choice of the antihypertensive agent can be personalized depending on the medical background of the person. *Beta-blockers* dilate the vessels to reduce the blood pressure. They are the second line of treatment for hypertension, especially for patients after a heart attack. *Angiotensin converting enzymes inhibitors* are suggested for diabetic patients. Clonidine, a medication that reduces the blood pressure by affecting the brain at specific sites (*central alpha-agonist*), may be used to treat hypertensive patients who have an intention to quit smoking or relinquish drug abuse[19]. Some *Calcium channel blockers* may have a favorable effect on angina. Since these agents and others may have side effects, the patient should be monitored on a regular basis. Combinations of low doses of two or more agents from different classes may minimize the likelihood of dose-dependant adverse effects. The key for a successful control of hypertension is adherence to therapy.

◆   ◆   ◆

In most cases, a healthy life style at a young age is a foundation for avoiding many medical problems in old age. Olivia Jones is a person who suffered from the consequences of smoking cigarettes and drinking alcohol during the early stage of her life. She will remain on blood pressure medications for a long period of time, and probably for the rest of her life because of her previous unhealthy behaviors. It is easy and imperative to avoid undesirable behaviors in order to keep our health at its best.

13

Never Ending Reality

Late one evening, my wife and I attended a defensive driving course. During the class, a familiar and important "life-saving topic" was presented. The instructor's strong message was absorbed deeply into my mind like a hammer firmly inserting a nail into a piece of wood. Upon leaving the class, as I tried to review the subject, the unforgettable memories of the past invaded my consciousness. They were all related to that special topic.

It was just before midnight when I went to bed. I rested my head on the pillow with the intention of falling asleep. But, unrestrained memories raided my serenity, interrupting my quiet mind. It was like a peaceful town invaded by a storm. Sleep, like an illusive "angel", was supposed to reinstate the tranquility in the town, but the gates were locked, barricading the angel's entrance. Therefore, I recalled my memories.

Reminiscences from the past belonged to the time when I resided in Israel, long before I entered medical school in that country. Until 1989, the first year of my emigration to Israel, I had never seen many of my family members who lived in that country. At the age of twenty-two, I moved to reside in Tel-Aviv, where my cousin, Ruth, lived. She was a native Israeli (Sabbar) and a soldier in military service at that time. As my hostess, she was willing to take me with her on most weekends to visit her parents who lived in "Hagalil", the north region of the country. Since I experienced tremendous difficulty trying to speak Hebrew, my communication with Ruth was mostly in English.

Ruth and I almost always traveled by bus to get to her parent's house. The road to their home was a narrow and winding one. The trip took about four hours. On each occasion the vehicle was usually packed with soldiers, local Israeli Jews and Arabs. This was a great opportunity for me to learn Hebrew from Ruth. It was also an enjoyable time to view the beauty of nature. The region was full of rolling hills and steep mountains. During the spring, a unique flower, "Kalanit", covered the valleys in a dazzling carpet of colors, mostly red with patches of purple. The excitement of the trip amused me so much that I would not perceive the passage of time! Once we alighted from the bus, we had to walk along a narrow road lined with trees, to reach at my aunt's house.

Ruth's mother, my aunt, was an immigrant who had lived in Israel for many years. Her house was always open to guests. For me, it was enjoyable to be with my younger cousins whom I had never met. They spoke in Hebrew, a language that I barely could understand at that time. My aunt was the only person who translated most of the conversations for me. In addition to my aunt's family, there was also a six-year-old boy living in the house. He was full of energy and did not miss any opportunity to dart around! "Who is this kid and what he is doing in this house? Why does my aunt love him so much and take care of him so nicely?" I asked myself. "The kid" was not alone. His thirteen-year-old brother was also free to come and go in my aunt's house. On occasion, I also saw a six-teen-year-old girl who had a wonderful relationship with my cousins. She actually lived in the house next-door. Interestingly, the two boys would disappear at night! Later on, I discovered they would go to sleep in the teenage girl's house! She was the boys' older sister! But, something was missing from the picture. "Where were their parents?" I asked myself.

As my aunt's guest, I was experiencing many difficulties acclimating myself to their customs and their language. I was young and did not have much self-confidence. I did not feel comfortable to inquire about those kids. However, after a few visits, I asked about the mysterious kids! Their story was so heartbreaking that, even today, the memory brings goose bumps to my skin! It was this disturbing memory that deprived me from falling asleep that night after returning from the defensive driving course. After many years, I was reviewing the lesson that I had learned from those kids. It was a lesson that thus far has been helpful in aiding me in protecting myself!

My aunt's other unusual neighbors were a "married couple", who were both in their late thirties. They did not have any children. After a while, I discovered the man was the second husband. It was obvious their relationship was somehow "different" for a second marriage. Again, I thought, who was I to question about the personal matters of people? However, curiosity was my motivation to discover more about these people. I thought something was different in their culture that I had missed. I was eager to gain more skills in order to survive in that society. What I learned could apply to any culture! I learned that the first husband was dead and the couple had decided to marry a year and a half after his death! I believe this was the first time I realized that death could change people's lives.

It took a few more visits before I finally asked my aunt about the full story of her "peculiar" neighbors.

"You know, Eddie! Probably, it was their destiny!" my aunt said with sadness in her voice.

"So! What happened to them?" I asked eagerly.

"One day, about three years ago, the parents of the three kids, and the next-door neighbor with her first husband went on a trip. They invited us to go with them, but we refused. We agreed to take care of the children until they returned. On the way home, the father of those kids was the driver." She took a deep sigh and stopped talking.

"What happened next?" I asked impatiently.

As my aunt kept looking at me, a teardrop slid down her cheek. Her starring at me was deep, without any blinking of an eye. I could realize she was going through painful emotions. As if her painful memories took her to a different world. Then, she raised her Lt hand and wiped her face.

"Once the water is poured down, you cannot collect it! Can you?" she asked.

"I guess not," I answered.

"Well, that's what happened to them," she said and continued, "You're already familiar with the winding road leading to our house. Unfortunately, the driver fell asleep behind the wheel, the car swerved and rolled down one of the hills along the road. Except for the woman, my neighbor, the rest of the three people were killed!"

"You mean that these kids are orphans?" I asked with despair.

"That's right! We agreed to take the responsibility of caring for the kids until they are grown. The girl will turn eighteen in two years. She will probably start working. The kids are lovely. We really enjoy them. We cannot be their parents, but as you see, with some help from the government, we are trying to give them what they don't have in their lives. And, the woman, as you know, remarried a year and a half ago," she explained.

This was a tragic story of a driver who was killed because of drowsiness. He died along with his wife and his neighbors. It was quite shocking to learn that someone's big mistake, a second of recklessness, might have a great impact and ominous consequences on the lives of others—a reality that never ends.

I rolled over in my bed. My eyes felt very tired, but the image of the little orphans from 20 years ago, kept me awake. The defensive driving instructor's words echoed in my head, "Don't drive when you are sleepy! Take a nap for 10–15 minutes and then drive." Finally, as my fatigue overcame the troublesome memories, my mind welcomed sleep—the angel of tranquility.

Fatigue

The next day, during my office hours, "fatigue" showed me its power in a humorous way! The safeguard of human alertness can be tricked easily. Once the desire for sleep emerges, it will have powerful effects, no matter where you are or what you are doing! You have to be sure that drowsiness does not occur while you are driving because of the possible injuries, loss of life, and other costs that take place.

It was around 2:30 p.m. I was ready to see my second patient of the afternoon. He was a new patient. I could hear his conversation with my secretary. Once I stepped out to welcome him, he stood up and extended his hand. Jon was an Oriental man in his forties, who was very fluent in English.

"Hello, doctor. Is it my turn?" he asked.

"Hello! Yes, sir. Please, come in."

As he sat down in the chair in the exam room, he said, "I'm sorry! I almost fell asleep in your waiting room. I just came in from Phoenix, Arizona this morning. I have not slept at all since last night!"

"I hope you will have a good sleep tonight when you go to bed!" I made a comment. "Well, how can I help you today?"

"I came here for a complete physical exam. I'm a cop! I'm going to retire in the next few months. I want to be sure that I'm OK."

"Do you have any medical problems?"

"As a matter of fact, yes! I had two car accidents in the last 6 months. I have a lot of neck and back pain. I'm also interested in knowing about my heart. One of my coworkers had to have thallium stress test to find out if he had some problems in the arteries of his heart! Do you think that I need such a test, too?"

Before I answered, I reviewed the questionnaire that he had filled out earlier in the waiting room. Then I said, "I don't know yet! According to what you answered on this form, it appears that you quit smoking many years ago. However, I see you drink alcohol socially. Is that a correct statement?"

"That's quite right!"

Then I changed the aspect of my questions. "You mentioned that you had two accidents. I'd like to know if at any time you were driving after drinking liquor?"

He quickly answered, "No!" After a short pause, he said surprisingly, "Yes! Actually yes! But this doesn't have anything to do with these accidents that I told you about!" Then, he explained how these accidents had occurred. Apparently, each one of them happened while he and his partner were chasing suspect cars. In neither of the cases was he the driver. Fortunately, each time he had his seat belt on! Knowing that an accident is serious, I listened to him carefully hoping to make him realize that I did care about what he went through. When he finished, he added, "No! No! I don't drink and drive!"

"That is good to hear!"

"Doctor! What about my heart? Do I need any tests?"

"Well, that's something else that we have to discuss." I asked him a few more questions and then I said, "Do you want me to proceed with the examination?"

"No problem, doctor," he answered and started to take his shirt off. As he turned around, he pulled a gun out from his shoulder holster. I have seen many different guns in my life. I even had to carry a gun from time to time when I was in the Israeli Defense Army many years ago, but still, the sight of a gun makes me anxious because of its destructive potential!

Jon placed the gun on the chair and sat down on the exam table. His exam was routine without any abnormalities. I asked his permission to obtain a resting electrocardiogram (ECG).

"What does the ECG show, anyway?" he asked, suddenly!

I smiled, and then said, "Good question! An ECG is like taking a picture of the heart. By tracing the electricity of the heart, one can see its structure and the rhythm. Occasionally, it might indicate whether there is a poor circulation to the heart muscle."

"OK, go ahead! I'm ready!"

On many occasions, I perform the ECG by myself. After Jon lay down, I put the electrode patches on his body. As I started to hook him up to the machine, he closed his eyes like many other patients do during this procedure. As I proceeded to enter his general information into the ECG computer, unexpectedly, I heard some strange sounds. I turned around to identify the source of the sounds. Surprisingly, It was the patient! He had fallen asleep and began snoring! A smile appeared on my face and, then, I carried on with the rest of the procedure.

Working with sensitive machinery can be occasionally problematic. This was the case when I tried to obtain the ECG on Jon. I had to adjust the patches and the electrodes back and forth to receive a precise reading. It was quite amazing that Jon's snoring became louder despite all of my manipulations! He was sleeping like a baby! When I finished, I let him sleep! Apparently my hard exam table was a very comfortable place for him! I looked curiously at his gun one more time, and I thought, "This guy has never seen me before. But, look how he leaves his gun unsupervised without any fears! What a power of trust in a physician! Or, is he really so tired that he forgot all about his gun?" Then, I silently laughed at my thoughts and at the high "volume" of snoring that Jon had been creating in the room!

Jon finally woke up after almost ten minutes of a pleasant nap. I was catching up with my notes. He looked more alert. We continued our conversation concerning the ECG and his heart. Jon did not realize but by allowing him to doze for a while, I was trying to prevent him from possibly having another car accident due to *the influence of sleepiness and drowsiness*. At least he became fresh enough to drive back home.

◆   ◆   ◆

On several occasions I felt tired or sleepy while behind the wheel of an automobile. In one instance, during my residency, the day after being on call all night, I was returning home in the afternoon. I felt very tired while driving on the highway. My eyes were so heavy that they began to droop, despite the fact that I had only ten more minutes to drive before arriving at home. The desire to fall asleep was so great that I had to pull over onto the service road. I parked my car in a safe place, pushed back my seat, and took a nap for more than an hour. Only then I did attempt to drive home. Surely, it was safe to drive after such a rest. I also learned to take a nap in the hospital after my night shift before I headed home. Ironically, I heard a similar story in the defensive driving course that I took. It was about a medical resident who had suffered several broken bones and a smashed face due to a road accident after a night on call! Luckily, he was alive!

◆   ◆   ◆

A human being needs to *rest* before performing any work, especially when there is a necessity for patience and precision. When someone sits behind the wheel of a car, not only his life, but also the lives of the passengers, other drivers, and pedestrians have to be protected. The individual's performance always can be improved after a good night's sleep or several hours of rest. People are killed every day because of different reasons. One of the major causes involves impaired driving under the influence of sleeplessness, alcohol, or drugs. It is possible to avoid these situations.

MEDICAL WISDOM

**Driving under the influence of <u>alcohol</u>, <u>drugs</u> and <u>drowsiness</u> is
an *attempt* to commit suicide and probably homicide.**

In 1999 and 2002, I attended two defensive driving courses. In the first one,
the highlight was on drinking and driving. In the second one, the emphasis was
not only on driving under the influence of alcohol, but also a major portion of
the message was geared toward drowsy driving. There has been a significant focus
on this subject in recent years. This prompted me to discuss this very important
issue.

An automobile is potentially one of the largest and heaviest killing weapons
that human beings have created. In 1999, in the United States, every 13 minutes
someone was killed as a result of a fatal vehicle crash, compared to one murder
every 34 minutes. This fact makes impaired driving the most frequently commit-
ted violent crime in America. Every 33 minutes, someone in the U.S. dies in an
alcohol-related crash. Every year, more than 17,000 people may lose their lives
due to alcohol related crashes. This number is slightly more than 40% of deaths
in all traffic crashes, making alcohol the single greatest factor in motor vehicle
accidents.

Now, imagine you have to drive with your eyes closed. What do you think
would happen? Either you go off the road or hit another car until you stop. It
requires a lot of courage to drive blindly. Unfortunately, every day, many people
do close their eyes and drive. They are "drowsy drivers". These are another group
of people, besides drivers under the influence of alcohol, who cause serious injury
to themselves and to others!

Each year, falling asleep while driving causes at least 100,000 auto crashes,
40,000 injuries and 1,550 fatalities.

These numbers are quite impressive! Sadly, the largest group affected by
drowsy driving is young men (ages 16–29), often "the brightest, most energetic,
hard working teens" whose crashes occur after midnight. The second largest
group is drivers over age 65, whose crashes tend to occur in early afternoon[13].

Drivers at risk

Get ready to lower your safeguards and fall asleep if you sit and drive long distances. You will easily get bored and may fall asleep quickly, especially if you are

already tired or under the influence of alcohol or drugs. The result could be a fatal accident or severe injury. The following drivers are at highest risk of becoming "drowsy drivers":

- Sleep deprived or fatigued (such as physicians and cops after night duties)

- Driving long distances without rest breaks

- Driving through the night (such as truck drivers), the early afternoon, or at other times when they are normally asleep

- Drivers who take medications that increases sleepiness, or drink alcohol

- Driving alone

- Driving on long, rural, boring roads

- Frequent travelers, e.g., business travelers

Warning signs of drowsiness!

To prevent a motor vehicle-related accident, once driving, you, as a motorist, should look for the warning signs of fatigue:

- Cannot remember the last few miles driven

- Drift from your lane or hit a rumble strip

- Experience wandering or disconnecting thoughts

- Yawn repeatedly

- Have difficulty focusing or keeping your eyes open

- Tailgate or miss traffic signs

- Have trouble keeping your head up

- Keep jerking your vehicle back into the lane

Solution

The only remedy for sleepiness is getting sleep! If you experience any of the above warning signs, please pull off into a safe area, away from traffic, and take *a brief nap*

(15–45 minutes). Scientific studies show that the common stopping remedies of getting out of a car briefly and engaging in some exercise or cranking up the radio will not counter drowsy driving[13]. Drinking coffee or other source of caffeine to promote short-term alertness might be helpful. However, it takes about 30 minutes for caffeine to enter the blood stream.

Another strategy to avoid an accident when you want to drive, but you are sleepy, is to get a ride from a family member, friend, or take a cab. Because young people are disproportionately represented in the category of drowsy driving fatalities, parents of teens and young adults are urged to let visibly fatigued friends of their own children sleep over, much as one would urge a visibly drunk person to avoid the road until their condition improved.

The attitude of drivers who fall asleep behind the wheel needs to be taken seriously. This behavior does not fit into the criminal category, but I believe the ruling will be changed. Drowsy driving can be as bad as drinking alcohol and driving! Dr. Allan Pack, Medical Director of the National Sleep Foundation of the United States, once said, "Motorists generally see drowsy or fatigued driving as an acceptable risk rather than a danger akin to drunk driving."

◆   ◆   ◆

Receiving a license to drive does not provide a person with a license to kill or to be killed. Whenever you feel that your driving i-3s impaired, remember that *arriving at your destination late is preferable to not reaching there at all.* As long as you are driving on the road, you can always stop or turn around. Once you are dead, there is no way to return to the road of life.

<u>Tips for a better sleep</u>

These are some ideas to improve your sleep. Each day, try to get regular exercise. Keep your bedroom quiet and at a comfortable temperature. Keep it dark enough. Use blinds or wear eye mask if needed. If you take medicines (including but not limited to sleeping pills) you should take them as directed by your physician. Keep the same routine each night to get ready for sleep (changing to nightclothes, checking doors and turning out lights). When you go to bed, relax your muscles. For this purpose, you can use an imaginary wave to begin in your feet and slowly works its way up to your head. Try to go to bed and get up at the same time every day.

To improve your sleep regimen, you should take a few more steps. Think of sleep as a nighttime activity. Do not nap during the day. Avoid exercise just before going to bed.

Do not engage in stimulating activities such as competitive game of cards or watching an exciting program on television just before bedtime. Try to stop these activities at least one hour before sleep. Caffeinated products, such as coffee, tea, chocolate, and caffeinated sodas may affect sleep adversely. Heavy meals and smoking disrupt sleep and, actually, so does alcohol. Remember: use your bed for sleep and sex. Do not read or watch television in bed. Do not use another person's sleeping pills. If you do not fall asleep within half an hour, it is better to get up and do some quiet activity. Then, return to bed when you are sleepy. Do not watch the clock or try to force sleep.

By using these steps your sleep will be deeper and healthier. You may need two to four weeks until you see the outcome.

◆   ◆   ◆

Slow down…

> *Well, I hope that this chapter has not made you sleepy because, I, your humble driver, like to take you to a new road with a fresh scenic view. From this point to the end of the next chapter, I'll raise a different subject—<u>humanitarian issues</u>. Therefore, keep reading if you intend to cover the next chapter, too. Otherwise, close the book and read it another day, when you are fresh.*
>
> *As an introduction, I would like to express a comment, which although not related to drowsy driving, is still related to fatigue and human existence. As a physician, I always seek to find venues to help people and prolong their lives. Unfortunately, in this world, there are some individuals who consider destruction a means to promote their interests. I mentioned in the beginning that, when I was in Israel, I rode a bus line on the weekends to journey to my aunt's house. Many years later, I traveled the same bus line to arrive at my military base camp while I served that country as a physician officer. Since the year 2000, Israel faced many suicidal terrorist attacks. In mid 2002, I heard that a bus had been blown up in that country as a result of a suicide bomber. When I investigated the case, I learned the bus belonged to the same line which I once used almost every day. You cannot imagine how lucky I feel that I do not have to use that bus anymore. At the same time, I experienced heart-wrenching pain because of the many people who lost their lives in that incident.*
>
> *Leading a nation is similar to driving an automobile. It requires special skills, precision, and the ability to reach the ultimate destination. In the Israeli-Palestinian conflict, people may kill their so-called "enemy" because they are simply "tired" of the long-term incongruity. The solution for human fatigue is simply a respite. Since the subject is close to my heart, I wish there would be a halt in the killing by granting rest to those exhausted people and the weary leaders of that region. Hopefully, this kind of action would bring peace. Amen!*

14

September 11, 2001

You have not made any mistakes! The previous page was intentionally left blank. It is my way of conveying the impact of September 11, 2001 and its aftermath. A blank page is a symbolic expression of my sorrow and respect for the loss of many human beings as a result of a terroristic attack on the World Trade Center. After the tragedy, my emotional distress level was such that I was paralyzed regarding the writing of any material for this book. For more than three months I also could not concentrate on my daily routine. Life appeared worthless, like the empty hollowness of an endless tunnel. My patients also suffered from an upsurge of anxiety for over three to four months. I was not spared by those feelings. I felt obligated to answer countless questions and deal with many of their concerns. All the while, I had to hide my personal emotions from those who sought comfort. My telephone line was jammed with conversations of people who called in for medications, seeking protective vaccines against bioterroristic chemicals, or simply a reassuring comment. All this was occurring during the time that I, myself, was suffocating inside because of constant apprehensive thoughts. As a physician, when I was confronted by a situation in which I ought to show leadership to my patients, I was also a student learning how to deal with biological terrorism and how to respond to many concerns adequately. The following stories are related to that time.

◆   ◆   ◆

<u>The first day after the attack</u>

The day after September 11, while I was still trying to comprehend the immense effect of the catastrophe on people, I received a telephone call from Emily Morgan, a patient of mine in her mid-sixties.

"Doctor Tabib," she said. "I know I have never asked you this, but I need to take some Valium. Please prescribe this for me! I'm desperate to take some. Please, doctor, please!"

"But, Mrs. Morgan, I cannot prescribe such medication without seeing you in the office," I answered passionately.

"Doctor, you don't understand! The son of one of my employees is missing! He worked in the Twin Towers. He is probably dead! I can't take it. Please, doctor. Would you prescribe some Valium?"

"Mrs. Morgan, I would strongly prefer to have a consultation with you in the office before prescribing Valium, especially because of the current situation!" It sounded as if I was repeating my explanation without understanding what she was going through. "You have never taken this kind of treatment in the past. This is not like regular medications. Valium is habit forming…" Before I could finish my sentence, I heard a click, indicating that she hung up on me!

◆   ◆   ◆

Two days later

On September 13, 2001, Thomas Schmidt, an old friend of mine, called me. We had the following conversation before any of the anthrax letters terrorized the nation.

"Ed, hi. Do you remember me?"

"Thomas!" I said surprisingly. "Is that you? It's been a long time since I've talked to you."

"I know. It has been about 5 years since we have spoken."

"It's a pleasure hearing your voice. How can I help you?"

"I'm sure you have heard about Cipro. You know what's happening. It's in the newspapers. It will come very soon. You'd better get some Cipro for yourself!"

"Cipro!"

"Listen! There will be anthrax or smallpox epidemics," he said with a trembling voice. "I think anthrax is going to be all over the place. It is written in the newspapers that Cipro is the treatment. Once the disease spreads, there won't be enough Cipro for every one! You and I have to better protect ourselves. You won't believe what happened next to my building yesterday. As you know, I work in Manhattan. A full squad of police and their cars were on the street. I don't know what they were doing, but I know that something is wrong in this country and they aren't telling us!"

"So, what do you want to do?"

"Ah...I don't know," he said apprehensively. "I talked to Lynn, my wife, last night. We decided to move out of New York! Maybe we'll go to Colorado."

"Really!" I said. "You really want to leave?"

"I'm almost positive. This anthrax is bad. I suggest you get Cipro. Get as much as possible! I have some and I need more. I'm most concerned for my children. They are small. They cannot take Cipro. They have to take a different antibiotic."

"Are you asking me to prescribe Cipro for you?"

"I'd appreciate it if you would. In return, if you or your family needs any help, please let me know. I can even provide you with accommodations in Colorado in case you choose to come with us. I'm serious!"

"You know, Tom! I think you'd better get a hold of yourself. I believe it's going to be OK."

"I wish you could help me! I'm desperate! I really need more tablets of Cipro! I'll have to get it from somewhere if you cannot prescribe it for me."

"Tom! An antibiotic is prescribed in case of an apparent disease. It is not used for prevention. I haven't heard about any case of anthrax yet."

"Ed, all I can tell you is that anthrax is coming! I suggest you get Cipro for yourself, your family and your parents!"

When Thomas and I finished our conversation, I thought, "Anthrax! When was the last time I saw someone with this disease?" Then, I answered myself, "Never!" Thomas's fear was so powerful that it caused me to immediately open a book and read about this subject. It was quite shocking to discover that there was no reliable vaccine against anthrax for humans. This probably was due to the impurity and complexity of the vaccine. Besides, using anthrax as a biological warfare agent has been known for years. I asked myself, "Why has no government authority done anything about protection yet?"

This was my introduction to the period of chaotic uncertainties following September 11, 2001. I had become familiar with the fear of anthrax a few days before this terror hit the United States. Thomas's prediction about anthrax turned out to be correct as the horror of this disease materialized. During the following days, while I had to support many of my panicked patients and struggle with their fears, my own level of anxiety continued to escalate. At times, I did not know what to tell them or how to behave. I felt I had to adhere to my physician's principles rather than yield to the unrealistic demands of people who requested prescriptions for antibiotics. Only the passage of time would reveal whether their fear of lack of protection was true or not. In addition, Thomas had mentioned the possible spread of smallpox! Would this prediction also become a reality?

◆   ◆   ◆

Three weeks later

Mahmood, an Indian man and a Moslem, was a patient in my practice. He worked in the World Trade center. Three weeks after the catastrophic collapse of the Twin Towers, he came to my office for a visit. He unfolded a miraculous story of how his coworkers and he himself were saved from the terrible disaster on that tragic day. Mahmood, in his early forties, was married and had 2 children. I could not imagine how his wife, Shahin, would have survived his loss if he had died.

Mahmood began his story speaking in a trembling voice. "I came down to the 54th floor to prepare for the meeting that had been scheduled with my bosses. I'm the fourth person in rank in my company. We had planned the meeting for nine o'clock on the 84th floor. I called upstairs, but no one answered. They were late. So, I continued working. Then, my telephone rang. It was one of my superiors. He said that he was going out for a smoke since the rest of the team hadn't arrived yet. I asked him about the meeting. He answered that I should wait."

"Did you stay on the 54th floor?" I asked.

"Fortunately, yes!" Mahmood replied.

"Then what happened?"

"A few minutes later, we heard this big boom! It was the other tower, on fire! We didn't know what was happening. I looked at my secretary. She said, "We are fortunate that the plane didn't hit our tower!" As we were looking through the window, suddenly we heard another big boom! This time it was our building that was hit. We all felt building shudder. All of us were frightened. Everyone began running downstairs! The hallway was packed with people. They were jumping from stairway to stairway to get out as quickly as possible! People were yelling. Once we got out, we ran away!" At this point, tears began running down Mahmood's cheeks!

Mahmood and I were silent for a moment. It was heartbreaking for me to see this man, at his age, crying. The event must have had a deep emotional impact upon him to bring up such a touching expression. I handed Mahmood a tissue to wipe his tears. Then, I asked, "What happened to your superiors? Weren't they on the 84th floor at the time of the accident?"

He smiled and shook his head gently. "They were lucky, too. One of them was late because he had a fight with his wife that morning! The other one overslept and missed the train! They never got near the buildings at all! It was just good fortune for all of us. Otherwise, we all would be dead."

"Wow!! What a fateful coincidence?"

"Believe me, Doctor Tabib! I'm lucky to be alive and to be sitting in front of you. I have two kids to raise. You know that I'm a Moslem! But, I don't understand why someone wants to kill us in the name of God."

"You are bringing up an important issue. Probably, you must have been thinking about this subject during the last few weeks."

"I'll tell you what it is. In Islam, whoever does not believe in Allah is called Kafar. This means that everyone who is not Moslem is Kafar because they don't call God, Allah. It is all about the name!"

"What is the verdict for Kafar?" I asked.

"He has to die!" he replied.

"But, does it really make any difference what we call God?"

"I understand this. But these tribes with radical beliefs don't!"

For more than half an hour, I sat with Mahmood listening to his emotional survival story and his religious commentary. He definitely needed a shoulder to cry on. I was lucky to have the opportunity to support him during the time of his despair. I was compassionate to his philosophy owing to my familiarity, to some extent, with Islam. In history, the sword was the answer for Kafar. Unfortunately, on September 11, 2001, a few suicidal pilots felt they were the messengers of Allah. They killed many innocent people!

With Mahmood, I had to break the confines of medicine and enter into the boundaries of religion and politics. My professors in medical school had taught me to be cautious when speaking about either of these subjects with my patients. These were sort of "forbidden" issues to be discussed! Not only on that day, but also on the days after my conversation with Mahmood, I felt that I had to break this taboo in my practice. By breaking the boundaries of such taboo, I was able to open my heart. This made it possible for me to view a new frontier in the understanding of human beings. Since then, many of my patients' emotional concerns have emerged due to having different groups of patients in my practice with various religious and ethnic backgrounds.

◆   ◆   ◆

The next three months

For a few months after September 11, 2001, like many other people in this country, I was in turmoil. My case was somehow different because I already had a background of experiencing terror as a young medical student in my native land, Iran. Members of radical Islamic groups had intimidated me because of my religion and my beliefs. Later in my life, during the late 1980's, I lived in Israel, where I was terrorized by daily news of Palestinian Arabs who stabbed Jewish people in the back. I learned to be vigilant if one of them would have marked me as a target.

During the aftermath of September 11, my feelings of distress and apprehension increased from day to day, especially when the threat of anthrax-tainted letters began. I purchased a few small masks for my secretary and myself to use when we were opening the mail. I was eager to learn more about anthrax in order to be able to answer my patient's questions. One day, at 7:00 PM, after my office hours, I rushed to the hospital to attend a seminar about the subject. Not surprisingly, the number of physicians and nurses participating was incredible. The entire auditorium was packed. During the ensuing weeks, I attended numerous medical grand rounds. Each time, the audience occupied all the chairs in the hall! As I learned more, I became more anxious.

In addition to myself, the entire medical community was also terrified as a result of the current situation in the country. While I became a student learning about bioterrorism, I still had to guide my patients who were victimized by the terror. I had to exhibit the brave face of "things would be OK" even though, at the same time, I was horrified myself. Eventually, the chilling thoughts of the present and the painful memories of the past brought me to the point of having to make crucial decisions about my life. My mind was occupied with the recollection of a philosophy book that I had once read many years ago. Jon Paul Sartre, a magnificent French writer, wrote this book, entitled "Existentialism". He believed in making choices in life. I felt that I had to select my pathway for the future. Since I already had the experience of being a "Wandering Jew", I thought I would have to move again. I had feelings of responsibility for my family. I would have to save them from anthrax, smallpox, dirty nuclear bombs and other weapons of mass destruction! Yet, I asked myself, "Where could I go?"

I was fortunate that an old friend learned about my fears. His simple and basic tale from Molavi, an ancient Iranian poet and philosopher, was like water being poured over a flame. The story was about a frightened man who went to King Solomon to plead for his own life! The man implored the wise king for help, "My Majesty, please, help me! I know that you can do wonders! Please, transfer me to India today!"

"Why India? What's wrong with our country that compels you to want to go to such a far place?" King Solomon asked.

"My Majesty, I have seen the angel of death today! This morning, he appeared before me in the street! He wore a black garment and a black hat. When he saw me his eyes opened wide! So, he caused me to be tremendously terrified! It was really frightening! I know that he wanted to take my life! So I want to go to India today to be safe. I don't think he will find me there!" the man explained.

King Solomon accepted the man's request. By using his extraordinary power, with a blink of his eye, Solomon transferred the man to India! Later that day, King Solomon himself met the angel of death. He inquired why the angel had frightened the man. The angel said, "I didn't try to frighten him. I simply showed my surprise at seeing him here, since I was told to take his life today in India!"

As I heard this story, my troubled soul became tranquil and peaceful. I came to the conclusion that destiny is not always in our hands!

◆   ◆   ◆

Six months later

Thinking about smallpox was frightening. Knowing that the Center for Disease Control (CDC) was preparing for a possible outbreak of this disease was even more alarming. The thought that a patient with a strange rash might be sitting in your waiting room was horrifying and unimaginable! However, that is the plight of being a family physician. Anyone, with any symptoms, may walk into the office.

One morning in my office, Barbara, my assistant, approached me. "You're going to have a new patient today," she said

"A new patient! That's good! I like to have new patients! Who is this one?" I questioned.

"I don't know! He just called and asked for an appointment for today! He said that he didn't feel well." Barbara stated.

"Another patient with a cold?"

"Probably!" she said.

"When is he coming in?"

"We had an opening at 10:30. So, I gave it to him."

A few minutes past 10:30, Barbara entered the exam room. Her body language was clearly an expression of her distressed mind. "Are you ready for the new patient?"

"Yes! Is there anything wrong?"

"He doesn't look good. He says that he has had a rash for a few days. Even I can recognize the rash on his face."

"A rash! Maybe it isn't as bad as you think. Ask him to come in," I said.

Alex was a European-looking young man in his early thirties. His body structure was muscular. He appeared very uncomfortable. His black hair was not combed properly, his face was unshaven, and his clothes were shabby. It looked as if he had just gotten out of bed. I saw that he was deeply troubled, as I noted that his hazel eyes were gazing around the room rather than looking directly at me. He stood in the room instead of sitting on the chair or the exam table. A reddish rash was apparent on his face. At that instant, a warning thought came to my mind, "Is this a case of smallpox?" Contrary to my customary greeting, I avoided shaking his hand because of the unknown and strange rash.

"Hello, sir. How can I help you?" I asked.

"I came in because of this rash. I had a little bit of it for the last 2 weeks. But, it has spread in the last 3 or 4 days. I even noticed that it appeared on my face. It's very uncomfortable, especially around my anus! It's painful every time that I sit."

I examined his face and immediately recognized this was not a "typical" rash. Something was different. I had to check the rest of his body to obtain a clue which would help me in making a diagnosis.

"Would you mind taking off your clothes so I can examine you?" I asked. While he was putting his shirt aside, I gently pulled out a pair of latex gloves from a box and put them on. As I evaluated his strange rash, I began questioning him.

"Do you remember if you ate anything different or unusual? Did you use any new material or even come in contact with another person with a similar rash?"

"No! Not that I remember any of these," Alex responded.

"I'm sorry to ask you a personal question. But, do you have sex?"

"Yes, I do," he answered as he looked away.

"Do you have sex with people that you don't know?" I asked.

"Yes!"

"You're telling me that you have had this rash for the last 2 weeks. Do you recall if you had any prior presentation, such as having a lesion, a few weeks ago?"

"Like what?" he asked.

"Do you recall if you had any ulcers on your genitalia?" I questioned.

"Not that I remember."

"Let me look at your hands," I said as I extended my arm to examine his hands. Through the latex gloves it was hard to feel the consistency of the rash, but it was flat and had a very obvious appearance on both palms. "Would you take off your shoes and socks?" I asked next. After Alex complied with my request, I proceeded to examine the soles of his feet. I discovered the rash was present there, too! Then, I thought, "Is this what I think it is? I have only seen this kind of presentation from medical text-books."

"Sir, I think you have a serious infection."

"What do you mean by serious?" he asked.

"I'm afraid that you may possibly have a rash from syphilis."

"Syphilis!" Alex challenged.

"You heard it right. This disease has three phases. In the second phase, a rash, similar to what you have, may develop," I explained.

Alex shook his head from side to side. He appeared confused. "So, what do you suggest I do?" he asked.

"If I'm right, you need to receive injections of penicillin. This is the preferred treatment for syphilis. But, before giving you a treatment, I have to make a definitive diagnosis. So, I need to do some blood tests on you."

"OK, do whatever you have to do," he said. He lay down on the exam table and then stretched his arm for me to draw the blood. As I picked up the needle, I asked, "Do you want to have a blood test for HIV, too?"

"No! I don't need that," he answered curtly while I was applying a tourniquet on his arm. Then, he turned his head toward the wall and suddenly said, "OK, do the HIV test, too!"

At the end of the visit, I asked Alex to be in touch with me the next day regarding the results of his blood test. Thus, we would plan his treatment.

During the evening, Alex was still very uncomfortable and in pain. He felt very suspicious about my hypothetical diagnosis. He decided to go to the emergency room of a large medical center for another opinion. As he walked in, the nurse directed him to the main waiting room. There were many patients near him. Upon examination, the emergency room physician diagnosed him with a "simple" rash. Alex was discharged with a prescription for oral antibiotic. He took home the prescription, but did not fill it, because it was late at night.

First thing the next morning, I called the lab to obtain the results of Alex's tests. They confirmed my clinical diagnosis of syphilis. This was a condition that is widespread in Africa, and apparently not so rare in New York, either!

"Syphilis!" I said to myself. I felt I had to inform Alex immediately. I picked up the phone and called him. Fortunately, I found him at home.

"Doctor, I went to the emergency room last night. They gave me a prescription for Amoxicillin. Do you think this is good enough?"

"Are you kidding me? This antibiotic is not going to help you at all! You need an immediate injection of penicillin! You'd best be followed by an infectious disease doctor. I'll call one of the physicians that I'm familiar with to make an appointment for you. I'll let you know right away."

Later, Alex received the penicillin shot from a well-known infectious disease specialist. After a few days, I had the opportunity to meet that physician. He said, "Ed, you did a fantastic job with the diagnosis on that patient with syphilis. These cases are very rare. I don't believe you'll see another case in your lifetime!"

I responded, "Thank you for the compliment. It was not an easy call. I'm simply wondering why the ER physician in that medical center misdiagnosed the case!"

"You're right. So I'll tell you what I did. I called the department head of the emergency room and criticized the physician who handled the case," he said.

This story may not be a perfect representation of the spirit of post-September 11. However, it is a starting point for initiating a discussion about a hypothetical patient with a rash resulting from smallpox. Let's imagine that such a person may wander around on the street. Later, he appears in a doctor's office to find out why he has the rash. Then, for whatever reason, he goes to the emergency room, which is congested with critical and non-critical patients. He might be told he has a "simple viral rash" or "food allergy" and then be discharged to home. The next day, he mingles with people. As a result of his activities, he is able to make hundreds of people sick with smallpox. Isn't that scenario similar to the case of my patient with the rash? Fortunately, although secondary syphilis has the potential to be contagious, this possibility is rare. The case of smallpox would be different. The United States of America is preparing for a possible attack of smallpox. Many hospitals are asking their medical and non-medical staff members to volunteer to receive the vaccine. These are the physicians, nurses, infectious disease specialists, and some ancillary service workers who staff the emergency room. Whether or not we use the smallpox vaccine for mass immunization is a question that remains to be answered in the future.

◆   ◆   ◆

History is for learning about and developing a new perception in life rather than simply knowing about a past incident. The events on September 11, 2001 were part of a painful history, which passed in front of our eyes. We all have memories of that day, which have given us a unique angle of vision about our community, our family, and ourselves. In larger perspective, those memories may guide us in reevaluating our relationship with people with diversified cultures who live in different corners of the globe.

Since the event of September 11, 2001, the fear of bioterrorism has launched a new perspective in medicine. For example, as a result, new medical school graduates, probably more than ever before, may learn additional information about an atypical rash. Some physicians might have modified their practice perspectives, as well. On occasion, religion and medicine might mingle, and patients may find a need to discuss their beliefs more openly. Every now and then, those patients are scared and need a compassionate individual to listen to them. In an ethnically diversified community, physicians may play an essential role model. By understanding the concerns of those people, physicians can be recognized as the messenger of peace.

Peace appears as a challenging goal in history to be achieved by the human being. For thousands of years, men have killed others or destroyed valuable structures because of political ideas, greed for land, or religious differences. Unfortunately, we have not learned that killing and destruction make people isolated from one another and do not produce unity. The terrorist attack against the civilians and the collapse of the World Trade Center can be recognized as a benchmark in the dark era of man's history that separated nations from each other.

To question the reasons behind the events of September 11, I like to go back to Mahmood, my patient, who spoke about God, a spiritual subject rather than a medical topic. His words could be an echo of the thoughts of many others. He blamed the differences in how we refer to God as a reason for the tragedy on September 11. At the time of his agony, he indirectly discussed the collision of conflicting beliefs. As he mentioned, in different languages, the Lord has various names. For semantic purposes, I will refer to "Him" as a male character. My vocabulary allows me to know him by many names, some of which have a specific meaning. In ancient Egypt, he was named Atone. Then, The Hebrews called him Adonye (the Master), and later, he received a new name by the same group of people, Elohim or briefly, El. Then, Moslem Arabs called him Allah. There is definitely a similarity between the expressions of "El" in Judaism and "Allah" in Islam! These two names are very close, but the groups of people who follow them are a world apart! This gap raises an important questions, "Does it really matter what we call the Lord?" These names and many others eventually led to the fundamental belief in a creating power of this gigantic universe. Therefore, let's preferably call him "the Creator".

What did "the Creator" want to achieve? I believe He tried to produce the "perfect" creature on the Earth. Without my entering into the philosophy of creation, He began working by shaping the first living organism, bacteria, and so far concluded by developing "the ultimate animal", the human being. This evolutionary process took million of years to achieve. The Creator wanted the best for his ultimate animal. Therefore, He made trees to supply oxygen for breathing, water for drinking, oil as the source of energy, soil for agriculture, and the sea for beauty. Besides those external resources, he rewarded the human being with an exceptional internal organ, the "brain". He provided the "ultimate animal" with the most complex brain for functioning. This creature, the human, has the ability to create, to build, to discover, to clone himself and, unfortunately, to cause destruction, or to kill his own species.

Destruction of buildings on both a large and small scale has been part of man's history. Historic architectures are examples of what human beings are capable. A simple example is the Coliseum in Rome. It is an enormous stadium with very tall brick walls, most of which are broken and in a state of rubble. This magnificent structure was built many years ago by the hands of Jews who were brought as slaves into the ancient Rome. Unfortunately, the Romans, themselves, destroyed it piece by piece a few hundred years later by taking bricks from the Coliseum walls for their own use. This is a small-scale example of how a human being could build and, then, destroy his own creation.

Besides destruction, killing is another ability of "the ultimate animal". By using his super power brain, a human is able to create the best machinery and then apply it in a wrong way. He is able to demolish buildings, flatten forests, cause air pollution, and even murder his own species! He performs these acts in a systematic fashion and in any fraction of time that he wishes. For example, during the six years of World War II, man was capable of killing more than 12 million people, among them 6 million Jews who were executed by gunshots or in gas chambers. In 1903, the Wright brothers had the idea of transporting people from place to place when they invented the airplane. However, I believe it never entered the minds of Wilber and Orville that their invention would be utilized as a tool for jeopardizing lives through hijacking, bombarding cities, or, in 2001, making New York's Twin Towers collapse, killing 2982 innocent people in less than 20 minutes!

Man carries out many destructions and killings of people that no other animal on the earth can accomplish. Then, ironically, he calls himself the noblest among the created beings! Did "the Creator" know his ultimate animal would become a "monster"? Does the ultimate animal ever learn from his own mistakes? Did humans realize that war would not solve the conflicts among nations?

It is a theory that dinosaurs were destroyed by an external force, such as the collision of a large meteor with the Earth. Are human beings the dinosaurs of today? Are we at risk of destroying ourselves because of an "internal force", which was created by us? In the second half of the Twentieth Century, during the cold war, the human being was intelligent enough to understand that attacking cities with atomic bombs could have been a simple game of tic-tac-toe which no one would win. Today, bioterrorism is the threat.

Bioterrorists believe that the dissemination of diseases, such as smallpox among the people of a nation, or the creation of terror by killing other humans, is the correct method to achieve their goals. They are deeply mistaken! A bioterroristic attack by smallpox outbreak may very well ravage their own nation, killing their own families, friends, and, even themselves. Thereby, it chases them from place to place. Today, this situation is different. Millions of people died as a result of this rapidly spreading infectious disease a few hundred years ago. Contrary to the present, at that time, there were no automobiles or airplanes. With the modern tools of today, it is possible that in less than three or four months, the disease could spread throughout a continent. Before we could comprehend what was happening, it would be all over the globe! It is simply insane to believe that by spreading smallpox, someone would think he had won a victory. The end result would have a disastrous outcome for every nation on the earth. The same consequences would occur by using any other weapon of mass destruction, biological or not, on a large scale. In the new millennium, there still are, unfortunately, some groups or nations who have forgotten that killing others is irrational, and "living" and overcoming disparities are the objectives of life.

The World Trade Center in lower Manhattan could not withstand the impact of the two large aircrafts because of its structural design. Perhaps, it was also destroyed due to a great disparity between the nations of the Western and the Eastern Hemispheres. Many people in the East think the people of the West have economically abused them. Among the Westerners, there are those who assume Eastern nations are lagging behind in technology and education. Such an attitude makes these two groups separate and total strangers rather than bringing them together. As Molavi, an ancient Iranian philosopher, once said, "We came to this world to unify people and not to disassociate them." Only "the brain" of the human being can develop the correct and proper venue for the coexistence of diversified civilizations. It is crucial that the mission of man be the preservation and protection of humanity rather than its destruction. The solution to the prevalence and continuation of peace between dissimilar nations is not killing, but learning about and understanding the cultural foundations of one another through dialog and respectful communication. Nothing, not religious beliefs, a piece of land, or political differences, are more important than life and existence.

I believe that good eventually prevails over evil. Mankind has a long history on the Earth. We can become "the *superior* ultimate animal" by preserving the heritage of the past and not destroying our future. It is preferable to use our energy to concentrate on conquering the unknown, inventing new tools, moving forward for better living, and promoting humanity, rather than thinking of methods to terrorize others. Life is already short. Let us not make it even shorter! We must learn from history and not repeat it.

MEDICAL WISDOM

It appears that there is an emerging need to protect civilians from bioterrorism. The Anthrax threats already caused terror in the United Stated. Smallpox, plague, tularemia, botulism and other biological weapons may also be on the way. Using rapid and effective actions in response to such attack can reduce the number of casualties.

Smallpox is a highly contagious disease found only in humans. It is caused by the virus variola. The disease may present itself in different severities from mild to serious. In a typical case, the symptoms may begin with fever, headache, weakness, vomiting, and, in some instances, diarrhea. It takes a week or two before smallpox lesions erupt. The rash first appears as minute red spots on the tongue and on the back of the roof of the mouth, along with small reddish spots on the face. The lesions spread in a circular fashion, involving the face, arms, trunk, and then the legs. Later, the rash in the mouth breaks down and releases large amounts of virus into the air. The reddish spots on the skin change to blisters (vesicular phase), and eventually become infected (pustular phase). The course of the disease lasts about 2 weeks. Then, crusts develop and the lesions heal, leaving scars.

Vaccination against smallpox goes back to the Tenth Century in China and India. During that time, it was noted that accidental exposure to smallpox by a scratch on the skin resulted in a less severe infection. Throughout the centuries, man has tried to find less risky ways of protecting himself from this disease. In 1796, Edward Jenner tried to prevent smallpox by administering a similar virus, called cowpox. In the recent century, the administration of another virus related to the smallpox virus, called vaccinia, controlled smallpox.

Endemic smallpox was eradicated from the United States in 1949. This led to the eventual discontinuation of routine childhood immunization by 1972, and the official announcement of its eradication from the globe in 1979. Since then, there has been no further vaccination for smallpox because of the possible side effects and fatalities from immunization. The adverse events might be life threatening in patients with reduced immunity, such as those with human immunodeficiency virus (HIV), individuals who undergo chemotherapy, and pregnant women. In the upcoming years, there will be enough vaccine available to inoculate every one in America, in case of a bioterrorist attack. It is sad to learn that over one thousand years ago humans fought to eradicate the smallpox virus from the Earth. Now, we have to struggle to prevent another insane human being from spreading this disease once again!

Anthrax can affect humans as well as animals, a factor that, contrary to small-pox, prevents its complete eradication. Except for the incidence of the "anthrax letters", which were distributed as a terrorist act in the United States in 2001, the disease is well controlled in this country because of an appropriate animal immunization program. Spores of anthrax, as offsprings of the bacteria, can live for 40 years. They can be found, for example, in the hair or wool of infected animals. Imported dolls and toys, decorated with infected hair or hides can be a source of infection.[14]

There are three types of anthrax. *Cutaneous* anthrax appears as a small reddish rash on the skin. Eventually, over a few days, it develops into a painless ulcer with a blackened background. This type of disease may develop as a result of contact with infected animals or animal products. *Gastrointestinal* anthrax occurs as the result of the ingestion of contaminated undercooked meat. It causes nausea, vomiting and severe bloody diarrhea, which may compromise the patient's life. *Inhalation* anthrax, the most serious form, is associated with severe shortness of breath and internal bleeding. This can be a deadly disease.

> It was a major concern for me when I had to deal with patients who came in close contact with anthrax in 2001. "Doctor, I work in the same building as Tom Brokaw. He got the anthrax letter today! Do you think I have to take the antibiotic?" a patient of mine asked. Obviously, her panic originated from the idea that the spores can travel through the air conditioning system of the building. Although that patient did not have to receive any antibiotics because she lacked symptoms, I did perform a nasal swab-screening test on her. A negative result was a source of comfort to her.

Isolation or visualization of the bacteria, through culture or staining, is the standard protocol for final diagnosis. Ciprofloxacin is the designated treatment in cases of exposure to the bacteria.

A word on sexually transmitted diseases

Many diseases are transmitted through intercourse or oral sex. Some of these are syphilis, gonorrhea, chlamydia, trichomonas, hepatitis B, papillomavirus (warts), HIV, and herpes virus. Early sexual intercourse in young females may also be a cause for developing cancer of the cervix (the neck of the uterus).

Although some sexually transmitted diseases have treatments, not all of them are curable. Infected persons may have long-term consequences from such contamination. They may end up being sick for the rest of their lives because of a moment of pleasure. Hepatitis B may cause chronic liver disease. HIV disease ends up with the potentially deadly condition of acquired immunodeficiency syndrome (AIDS). Pelvic Inflammatory disease, an infection of the female reproductive system, is caused by bacterial infection. This may result in infertility, chronic pain, or pregnancy outside of the uterus.

Abstinence from sex is the safest method for preventing sexually transmitted diseases. It may sound old fashioned, but self-restraint from sex as long as possible, even until marriage, reduces the chances of contracting sexually transmitted diseases. During this period of being celibate, masturbation might be a solution for sexual satisfaction. The basic lesson for heterosexual partners and male-homosexual relationships is to use a condom. This can be the easiest and simplest tool to use in order to avoid many of those diseases.

◆   ◆   ◆

Emily Morgan, the patient who asked for Valium, eventually obtained her pill from a friend. As a result of September 11, 2001, Mahmood eventually quit his job and four years later, he was forced to move to a southern state. Thus, I lost him and his family as my patients. Alex came back to visit me a year later for an attack of shingles on his face. Since then, I have not seen him. For hopefully a more peaceful world, Mr. George W. Bush and Toni Blair remained in power and were reelected. And, I kept residing in New York and expanded my practice to concentrate on healthy living.

15

Live Longer and Stay Younger

Since so many unexpected events occur every day in this world, we are lucky to survive. Being well informed and equipped with certain knowledge allows us to remain healthy. There are many situations, which put our lives at risk of either becoming ill from disease or injured as the result of accidents. Fortunately, many of these conditions are preventable. In this chapter, I point out many of the steps you can take in order to protect yourself from environmental hazards and undesirable health habits. The following subjects will be discussed:

I)   Stress and Coping Mechanisms
II) Accident Prevention
III) Preventive Aspects of Dental Care
IV) How to Avoid Diseases
V)   Love and Relationship

I) Stress and Coping Mechanisms

I perceive the basic human needs to be comprised of three layers. The *first layer or elemental needs* are quenching thirst, satisfying hunger, eliminating bodily wastes, and resting well. The *second layer* accounts for the enjoyment of the five senses: hearing, sight, smell, taste and touch. The *third or advanced layer* is related to the satisfaction of the higher functions of the brain such as desire and emotion. In this last category, we can find fulfillment of sexual desires, achievements, love, respect, and forming relationships.

When the elemental necessities for a human being are properly fulfilled, the individual then has the tools required to enjoy life. However, it is also the nature of the human being to satisfy the second and the advanced layers of needs. Any interruption, damage, or loss in any one of the layers may lead to *stress*. For example, deprivation of sleep from the first layer, hearing impairment from the second layer, loss of a loved one, an enthusiasm for obtaining a higher education, or achieving financial security from the third layer, all signify the creation of stress at different degrees and its many health related by-products. Some of the important end-results are summarized in figure 1.

In most instances, we cannot alter the course of a stressful situation. These taxing conditions may develop because of the loss of or change in a valuable object, a person, or a relationship. The most stressful events arise due to the separation from a close person, such as with the death of a spouse. Other high-tension producing situations include divorce, marital separation, time spent in jail, or the death of a close family member.

> *Jordan, a 70 year-old man, came to see me for a complete physical exam before traveling to his native country to visit his family. He had planned the trip for months. He was very enthusiastic about uniting with his family members, especially his close brother, whom he had not seen for many years. His medical conditions, which included high blood pressure and hypothyroidism (under-active thyroid gland), were stable with the use of medications.*
>
> *Upon arrival at his destination, Jordan discovered that his brother had passed away about a year earlier. No one had informed him, fearing that the news would cause him to be emotionally upset. After receiving the news, Jordan became very distressed. His blood pressure rose to an abnormally high level of 200/100. Then, his physical condition worsened. He had to be hospitalized for congestive heart failure and a dangerous irregular heartbeat, called atrial fibrillation. Jordan remained in the hospital for 10 days.*
>
> *Upon his return home, he came to my office for a follow-up visit. He cried hard! He was not only depressed, but also anxious and mentally unfocused. He needed new medications and ample amounts of compassion and support. I wonder how the stress of learning about the ever-lasting separation from his brother played a role in Jordan's scenario.*

By using the right coping mechanisms, we can reduce the level of stress or bypass some of its harmful effects. In order to reduce stress, one may choose an unconventional pathway, such as seeking refuge under the shelter of drinking alcohol, eating "comfort" foods, reckless spending, or gambling. These actions, or similar ones, do not decrease the level of stress or anxiety. They only put a person in a vicious cycle by amplifying the original stressful situation! Coping mechanisms to ward off stress-producing factors can be utilized in a regulated and rational fashion. These are illustrated in figure 2.

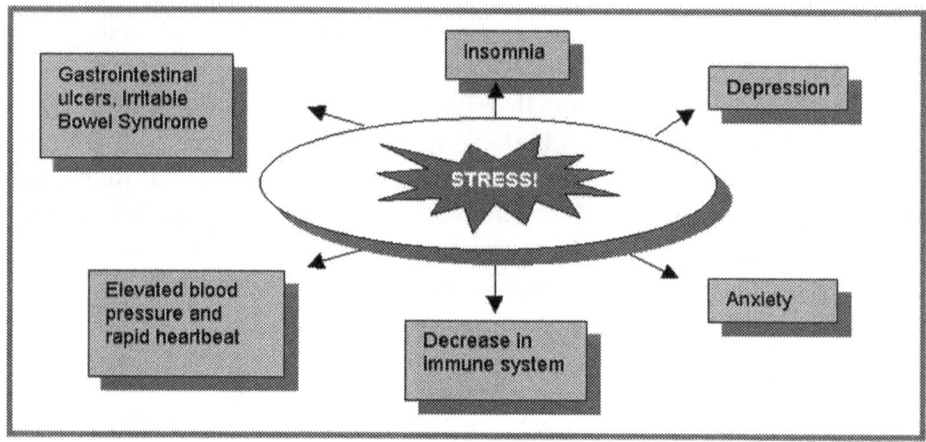

Figure 1—Medical and health-related consequences of stress

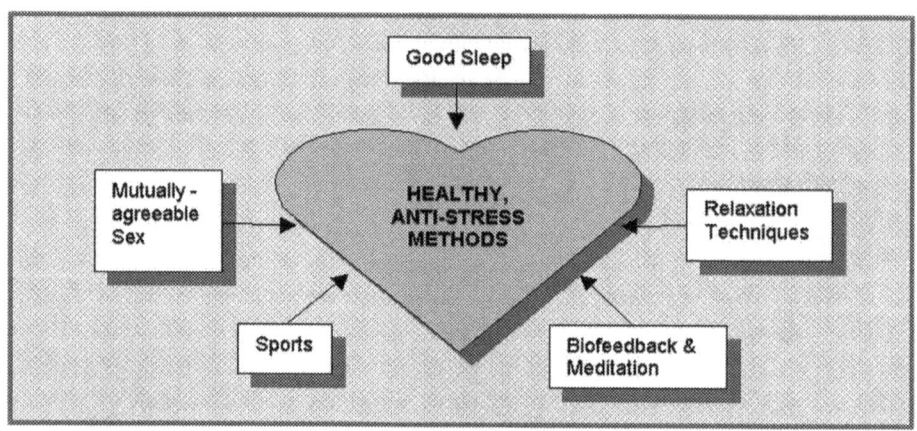

Figure 2—Coping mechanisms for stress

In every stressful situation, always ask yourself whether you have satisfied the elemental needs of living. An affirmative answer may grant you a comfort zone. *A happy life, with a minimum amount of stress, may prolong your existence on the Earth.* The assimilation of the famous idea of "no worries", on a daily basis, may help you follow a peaceful and longer life.

II) Accident Prevention

For children and young adults, the leading cause of death is accidents. Avoiding stress may reduce the risk of accidents. Following certain conditions to create a non-stressful environment may reduce the risk of injuries.

There are conditions that may lead to accidents. Change or instability in a person's environment may raise the level of anxiety, thus increasing the chance of accidents. Children may not be able to fully express themselves in a stressful situation. Instead, they may engage in activities that put them at risk of injuries. The death of a family member, maternal or caregiver illness, recent change in the caretaker, relocation or vacation time, or a tense relationship between parents are examples of variations in the children's environment that puts some strain on them. Caregiver preoccupation—rushed or too busy—is another example of an unstable condition. Saturday was found to be the worst accident day, and 3 to 6 PM were the worst hours. Parents and educators must also watch hyperactive children since they may not realize the dangers of certain games.

For safety of yourself and your children, remember the following:

1. Don't remain hungry or tired! Injuries occurred more frequently during the hour before a scheduled meal, in the late afternoon, or before bedtime.

2. When driving your car, remember to use a *seat belt* for yourself and your children *at all times.*

3. Supervise your children in water, in the street, or while playing in the yard.

4. Wear a helmet during high-speed games, such as roller-skating, ice-skating, or bicycling.

III) Preventive Aspects of Dental care

It has been said, "If you take care of your teeth, they will take care of you!" Teeth are one of the most important parts of our body since they are the shiny entry gates to the digestive system. It is imperative to keep them healthy for as long as possible.

As parents, we are responsible for the care of our children's teeth. In infancy and early childhood, after the ages 1 or 2 years old, doctors discourage parents from bottle-feeding babies just before bedtime. Bottle-feeding in bed not only may cause dental caries, but also may lead to serious ear infections.

Fluoride is an important element needed during the period of tooth formation. Tests show the ingestion of water containing the optimum concentration of fluoride has consistently resulted in a 40% to 60% reduction in dental caries. It is recommended to take multivitamins containing fluoride if your water supply has a low concentration of this important element. Oral administration of fluoride should begin soon after birth and continue until the ages of 12 to 14 years. Having a diet rich in calcium, plus related nutrients, including phosphorous, magnesium, and vitamin D, is essential for developing healthy teeth. Poor dentition in elderly people may signal osteoporosis. The presence of this disease signifies the need for further evaluation by having a bone density scan.

Parents are the role models for children. Tooth brushing, at least 2–3 times a day, for duration of 2–3 minutes, is a very important step in maintaining oral hygiene and gingival health. Every night, as you brush your teeth, teach your children how to brush theirs. Because of its simplicity, the use of short, horizontal, scrubbing strokes is a desirable method that can be readily mastered by both the child and parents. The application of *plastic sealant* to caries-susceptible pits and fissures of teeth is a recent advancement in the prevention of dental caries.

IV) How to Avoid Diseases

As a physician, besides prescribing the proper medication, I find myself helping patients to choose the appropriate diet or method of preserving their physical condition. Therefore, I have decided to provide you with some dos and don'ts in table 1. This list may help you to cope with some common medical situations you might encounter throughout your life. Most of these conditions have been discussed in different chapters of this book. Some circumstances are discussed here as special considerations.

The wonders of laughter

Laughter and happiness may increase the body's immune system levels by lowering stress. Looking at life in a humorous way may increase the productivity of your work. It is even suggested that laughter increases the length of life. Physicians may reduce the tension associated with an office visit and develop a better rapport with their patients when they amuse them with the power of laughter.

Many years ago, during the last few weeks of my residency, I requested to work morning hours with one of the attending-teachers. "Be in my office at 9:00 o'clock," she said. The next day, I arrived at her office 5 minutes before 9:00. Except for her secretaries, no one else was in the office. As I waited for her, my attention was drawn to a four-by-four inch, thin reference book that sat on the shelf of her library collection. It contained every piece of para-medical information that a physician needed to be a success. I read it through, and for some unexplained reason, I memorized many of its passages. I was almost finished with the book when the attending teacher appeared in her office at 20 minutes after 9:00. During those twenty minutes, I had enough time to learn several essential lessons concerning the managing of patients.

One of the lines of that book read, "If you want to hear only medical complaints from your patients, that is all you will hear from them." Since then, with my patients, I listen to their medical concerns and also open my heart to their stories. I talk to them about their beliefs, politics, religion, family, and other issues. Above all, I also laugh with them. I discovered laughter to be one of the best and easiest ways to connect to people. Some of my patients are so accustomed to the idea of telling jokes that they do not leave my office before doing so. The following medically related comic stories might bring a smile to your face, too. All of them are from or about my patients. Don't be shy. Read them all!

1. *An elderly man went to see a doctor. The doctor said, "I have two kinds of news for you. One is good and the other one is bad."*

    The patient said, "Well, tell me the bad news first, and then the good one."

    The doctor said, "The bad news is that you are dying."

    The patient, raising his eyebrows, then asked, "If this is the bad news, what is the good one?"

    "The good news is that you have Alzheimer's disease. You'll forget the bad news before you leave my office!"

2. *An 83-year old patient of mine came to me and said, "Doctor, you got to help me."*

    "What happened to you?" I asked.

    "I have become forgetful. I believe I've gotten Alzheimer's disease."

    "Don't worry!" I said. "Patients with Alzheimer's don't complain about their disease. Therefore, you probably don't have it."

    Six months later, and two days after his 84th birthday, he returned to my office and said, "Doctor, I found out what was wrong with me! I'm suffering from a new syndrome—Birthritis!"

    "What is this?"

    "I had too many birthdays!"

3. *One of my patients, in his late 60's, was living in New York. He had 4 grown children and 10 grandchildren. Two years after his wife died, he began a relationship with a lady who lived in Florida. His children did not welcome the new relationship, saying that she symbolized their late mother. My patient would not tolerate his children not agreeing with his new relationship. One day during the winter, he decided to travel to Florida to be with his lady-friend. As a matter of courtesy, he asked his children to join him. The children responded, "Well, that is OK, dad. We'll eventually be there, but probably in the summer-time."*

    My patient, who actually wanted to be alone with his friend, said, "No problem at all! That is a great timing! Because by then, we will be back in New York!"

4. *Two hunters were in the wilds of New Jersey. Suddenly, one of them collapsed. The other one panicked and anxiously called the emergency line.*

    "Operator, my friend had the shakes and then collapsed. I'm afraid he's dead!" The man said in horror.

    "Calm down, please. First be sure that he is dead!"

    The operator heard nothing but silence on the telephone line for a moment. Then, she heard a gunshot. The man's voice returned on line and he said, "OK! He is definitely dead. Now what?"

5. *I heard the following joke from an elderly woman who was a resident of a nursing home. She was blind because of macular degeneration, but her spirit was alive and healthy.*

    A woman entered a doctor's office for an examination. The doctor said, "Ma'am! Please, go to the room and take off your clothes!" The woman turned around and said, "You first!"

How to prevent kidney stones

Several factors may increase a person's chances of developing kidney stones. Male gender, increasing age, diet, geographic factors, some diseases, and certain medications are among the risk factors for kidney stone formation. The increased intake of protein, salt or oxalate, and the decreased intake of calcium and fluids may also increase the risks of stone formation. The restriction of consuming dairy products to reduce calcium intake is no longer appropriate advice. In fact, groups of men and women with the highest calcium intake have been shown to have nearly one-half the probability of developing stones as compared to groups with the lowest intake. Calcium citrate is the preferred agent for calcium supplementation in both men and women who have a risk of stone formation.

At least 8 to 12 ounces of fluids should be ingested at bedtime to lower urinary concentration, which usually occurs during sleep. Water is the preferred beverage. Citrus juices, such as orange juice—with or without calcium—also appears to diminish the risk of stone formation.

Avoiding the consumption of nuts, chocolate, dark green leafy vegetables, tomato sauce, and jams, containing high amount of oxalate, may also reduce the risk of stone formation. The ingestion of large quantities of salty foods or high amounts of protein (such as poultry and meat) may increase that risk. In certain group of patients, physicians may prescribe diuretics (water pills), such as hydrochlorothiazide, to prevent the recurrence of kidney stones.

> *Gas pain or kidney stone?*
>
> *Late one afternoon, Norman, a 30 year-old man, called me on the phone because he had abdominal pain.*
> *"I have this pain in my belly that I can't get rid of. It's all gas. You have to see me today!"*
> *I could not ignore his demanding voice. "OK, come in now," I said.*

As soon as Norman entered the office, I noticed that he held his hands over the right lower side of his abdomen and walked in a bent-over position. I said, "You have a kidney stone!"

"Do you really think so?" he asked.

"According to the way you behave, it looks like the correct diagnosis. But, tell me, is your pain constant or does it come and go?"

"It's constant."

"Constant? Well, this is not typical regarding a kidney stone. All right! Would you lie down on the table for examination?"

As soon as he rested on the table, he said, "Hay, you see, the pain is gone! I told you it was gas!"

"So, the pain is not constant. Are you cured or did my magic hand relieve your pain temporarily?"

"I really feel better. What do you think I should do now? Do I have to leave it alone or..."

Norman could not finish his sentence. He suddenly appeared to be in agony, "...Ah, It's back again. It's back!"

After I finished examining him, I said, "I think I'd better check your urine specimen."

The results of the urine test made me confused. There was no indication of blood in his urine—supposedly a hallmark in making the diagnosis of a stone. "What kind of kidney stone is this?" I thought to myself. "It doesn't show any blood on the urine test strip. Am I missing something or what?"

"Norman! You have all the indications of having a kidney stone, but your urine specimen does not fully support it! I'd rather work you up in the hospital. You might need more advanced evaluation."

I called an ambulance to take Norman to the hospital. His urine test in the emergency room also did not show any trace of blood. A CT scan of the abdomen, however, showed a very tiny stone located in the upper part of his right ureter (the small tube that connects the kidney to the bladder).

Norman remained in the hospital for 3 days. During this time, he had to undergo a procedure to remove the stone.

This story illustrates that an initial clinical impression might be superior to some basic diagnostic tests. An advanced test may be needed to support the initial judgment and providing more information about the patient's condition.

Table 1—Combat medical conditions with life style modifications

Condition	Not Recommended	Recommended
Acne	Oil-based makeup, hair gels and sprays, suntan oil, stress, anxiety, squeezing and picking at blemishes, and scrubbing the skin hard.	Keep your skin dry.
Constipation	Foods high in fat and oils (such as heavy creams, butter, and sausages), cola, carbonated drinks, chewing gum, "gassy" foods (such as beans and cabbages), and anxiety.	High fiber diet such as whole wheat bread, fruits with their skin, especially prunes.
Diarrhea	Milk and other dairy products (plain yogurt is controversial), raw vegetables, fruits with their skin - for duration of 5-7 days - coffee, alcohol, smoking, and anxiety.	Take plain yogurt, tablets of Acidophilus or Bacid, boiled vegetables, bananas, and soup.
Gout	Meat, poultry, fish, spinach, asparagus, mushrooms, beans, peas, oatmeal, rye bread, cereal, whole wheat, and alcohol.	Take low fat dairy products, water, and high starch/ vegetarian diet. Try to loose weight.
Heart Disease Hypertension Diabetes Mellitus	Highly salted, fatty and sweet foods, smoking, and alcohol.	Take normal or low salt, low fat, low sugar diet, and exercise.
Ulcer of the esophagus, stomach and duodenum Heartburn	Alcohol, smoking, spicy foods, Vitamin C, coffee, tea, cola beverages, chocolate, peppermint, acidic foods (such as tomato and orange juice), and aspirin.	Take blended high protein diet for a few weeks after the diagnosis, and then regular diet. Raise the head 4-6 inches, in case of heartburn, when lying down.
Kidney stones	Nuts, chocolate, dark green leafy vegetables, tomato sauce, jams containing high amount of oxalate, salty foods, and ingestion of high amount of protein (such as poultry and meat).	Take 8 to 12 oz of fluids (at bedtime). Take calcium citrate.
Osteoporosis	Smoking, meat, poultry, and alcohol.	Take calcium supplement with vitamin D, and exercise regularly.
Rosacea	Hot liquids, alcohol beverages, spicy foods, sun, and extreme of temperatures.	
Urinary tract infection (females)	Douches, bubble bath, tampons, and tight pants.	Take cranberry and blueberry juice, and plenty of water. When using the restroom, wipe and wash from front to back. Urinate after sex.

GERD (acid reflux disease)

In recent years, GERD, or gastroesophageal reflux disease, has become a common term used by patients in many medical practices. Technically, it is the return-flow of acid from the stomach to the esophagus. This acid can cause pain in the upper part of the abdomen *(epigastric pain)*, commonly called *heartburn*, and it may or may not be associated with chest pain. The name of the symptom is very misleading. However, if the pain actually originated from the heart, it would be called angina. Interestingly, both of these symptoms might occur immediately after a meal, making the diagnosis even more difficult, especially in elderly people or in smokers. In many cases, the back-flow of acid may cause a *chronic cough*, similar to cases of early asthma. In one case, a patient of mine suffered from hoarseness *(laryngitis)* when he awoke every morning. A recurrent acid reflux will cause severe damage to the lower part of the esophagus, leading to *difficulty in swallowing (dysphagia)*. Obviously, these symptoms will vary in severity in different patients.

On a daily basis, GERD may present itself in up to 7 percent of the population. Many others, especially overweight people and smokers, may experience this condition at least once a month. Some medications, such as non-steroidal anti-inflammatory drugs (Advil®, Motrin®, ibuprofen, etc.), bisphosphonates (alendronate, risedronate, etc.—a type of medications for treatment of osteoporosis), tetracycline (a kind of anti-microbial agent), and β-blockers and calcium channel blockers (medications for heart disease and hypertension), may aggravate the acid reflux.

Dietary measures are outlined in table 2. Some medications, as first-line therapy, are helpful in the treatment of acid reflux disease after life style modifications. These agents, essentially, reduce the stomach acidity and decrease the risk of damage to the internal lining of the esophagus. Over-the-counter antacids (Maalox® or Tums®, etc.) or H_2-receptor blockers—acid blockers—(Zantac®, Pepcid AC®, etc.) are adequate as initial remedies. A more aggressive management to reduce the acidity of stomach secretions is the use of a higher strength of H_2-receptor blockers, or taking proton pump inhibitors (PPI's). Omeprazole (Prilosec®) was the first agent in the category of PPI's that was introduced to the market many years ago. Today, several similar products are available. Regardless of the cost, these agents have comparable outcomes with tolerable adverse effects. A 6-week treatment with PPI's as the therapy for GERD is recommended. An aggressive evaluation, such as upper endoscopy, is considered if the treatment fails. In many cases, a long-term maintenance therapy might be required.

For two years, seventy three-year-old Anthony was known to have a very mild disease of one of his coronary arteries (the arteries that supply blood to the heart muscle). He was faithfully compliant with his heart medications. When he left the country on business, he began to suffer from frequent belching and pain in the upper part of his abdomen. While abroad, he underwent an aggressive treatment for GERD, which included an upper endoscopy to visualize his esophagus and stomach. He indeed was found to be afflicted with acid reflux disease. He took treatment with PPI as prescribed. Nonetheless, he had no relief from his discomfort.

Upon his return to the United States six months later, he visited his cardiologist, who recommended an angiography to examine his coronary arteries. In this procedure, a thin long tube is inserted through the groin up to the heart. An injection of a dye maps the inside of the coronary arteries and indicates any obstruction in them. The results of the test showed that the condition of Anthony's coronary arteries had become worse. He was actually on the verge of a heart attack! He underwent treatment with a balloon angiography and the insertion of a short spring (stent) inside of his diseased artery. The relief of his symptoms was immediate.

The presence of one disease does not necessarily eliminate the risk of another one!

Sun and its effects

It is essential for our skin to be exposed to sunlight to manufacture vitamin D. This vitamin helps our bones to develop and be protected. Throughout the day, ten to fifteen minutes of sun-exposure is adequate for the skin to provide a sufficient amount of vitamin D. Beyond this length of time, the sun may cause harm to the skin or to the eyes. Lengthy exposure, especially at an early age, may cause even more severe damage. Skin cancers, thickening of the skin, and formation of cataracts of the eyes are among common problems resulting from prolonged exposure to the sun.

Fisherman

One summer-afternoon, Jeffery and his wife came into my office. He was an early-retired, mildly obese, bearded Caucasian man, in his mid fifties. His main complaint was a cough. But, I could not ignore noticing his deep suntan as he walked into my exam room.

"Where did you go to get such a tan?" I asked.

"I went fishing last week," he answered quickly. "I have a yacht. I go fishing a few times a week. I've been doing this for the last 10 years. Maybe one of these days, you can come with me, too!"

"Thank you, Jeff. Maybe, one day, I will. Meanwhile, let me examine your lungs because of your cough."

As he pulled up his shirt for me, I saw a very tiny black dot on his lower back, just above the level of his belt. As he leaned forward, his obese abdomen pulled his belt further. This maneuver enabled me to see two more dots. I became curious. I asked him to open his belt. Then, I discovered a bunch of black spots.

"How long have you had this discoloration?" I asked.

"Which discoloration? I can't see my back," he replied.

"You are right, but I can! You have a strange mole on your back. You'd better take care of this immediately!"

The next week, Jeffrey underwent an extensive removal of the skin of his lower back. He had malignant melanoma, a very dangerous skin cancer. In Jeffery's case, his cancer developed due to prolonged sun-exposure as he repeatedly bent over in his yacht to catch a fish. Over a few years, this kind of cancer may be deadly since it tends to invade the skin and other organs.

For a long time I lost track on Jeffery. Five years later, I held a conference in a senior citizen center. At the end of the session, a nice lady approached me and said, "Do you remember me? I'm Jeffery's wife."

"How could I forget you?" I answered. "How is Jeffery doing?"

"Thanks to you he's still alive and healthy and enjoys his fishing."

Once I heard the good news, I was happy that, five years before, I was curious enough to see what was going on under Jeffery's belt!

Watch your legs!

After two years of noticing an ulcer on his wife's leg, a man convinced his sixty-five-year-old wife to come in and evaluated by me. She indeed had a 5 by 5 cm ulcer on the side of her leg. There were no signs of infection.

"Why didn't you come in earlier?" I asked.

"I'm scared of doctors!" she replied.

As I asked more questions, I learned she liked to wear skirts since a young age. This practice caused her legs to be exposed to the sun for many years. She ended up with a large incision and a skin graft to remove a basal cell carcinoma, a benign cancer of the skin[21]. She could have been saved from this big procedure if she had come in earlier.

To protect your skin from long exposures to the sunlight, use a sunscreen with sun-protective factor (SPF) of 15 or higher. Choose a brand that protects against Ultraviolet A and B radiation. With prolonged sun-exposure, multiple applications of sun block are recommended during swimming or any other activities. Don't skip applying sunscreen on any exposed part of your body, including your ears, lips, nose and hands. A hat with a large brim may be helpful to protect your face, too. Using Ultraviolet-resistant sunglasses, from an early age, may also prevent cataract formation. The key element to minimize any sun damage is to avoid prolonged sun-exposure.

Vaccination

Vaccination, a method for preventing illnesses, introduces a weak form of a disease into the body. Most of the children in the United States receive immunization from their pediatricians. Somehow, once people pass the age of 25 years, many of them forget they need a continuation of vaccination through adulthood.

Diphtheria-Tetanus vaccination is needed every 10 years. *Pneumonia vaccination* is indicated for people with chronic diseases or after the age of 65. This vaccine is recommended once or twice during a lifetime, based on the primary administration and the medical background of the patient. This vaccine either protects a person from becoming ill with a common bacterial pneumonia or, at least, reduces its severity in the case of contracting the disease.

Hepatitis B, a serious liver disease, may lead to severe liver damage, such as cancer or cirrhosis. It is mandatory to receive *Hepatitis B vaccine* right after birth. It is also indicated for health-care professionals, patients with chronic diseases, or anyone who requests it.

Influenza, a viral disease, causes a severe form of pneumonia with possibly deadly consequences in the elderly. Upon contraction, you may experience a very high fever and chills. These symptoms may disable you for a few days. Therefore, *flu vaccination* is recommended for every one who does not have any contraindication to it. Since the virus changes from year to year, a new vaccine has to be injected into the muscle annually. A nasal form is also available for certain groups of people. This inhaled vaccine contains a live, but weakened, influenza virus. At the present time, Center of Disease Control and Prevention guidelines suggest this vaccine for use in healthy, non-pregnant persons between 5–49 years old.

Herbal medicine

In today's medicine, the knowledge of homeopathy has become part of the routine management of patients. The Food and Drug Administration has not approved some herbal products due to the fact they may contain impurities. There also is no hard evidence of their effectiveness. The following list contains information about some herb products and extracts.

Echinacea, at the dose of 800 mg per day, can be used to treat colds, wounds or other irritations, and HIV disease. One study, which was done on children, did not show any advantage of taking this herbal remedy over placebo, and it could be associated with an increased risk of rash[24].

Feverfew is used in the prevention or treatment of headaches, migraines, and osteoarthritis.

Garlic is claimed to lower cholesterol and blood pressure. Animal studies have been conducted on its cancer prevention activity. The dose is usually 600–900 mg per day. The active ingredients are found in fresh garlic or enteric-coated tablets (Kwai), but not in deodorized or dried products.

Glucosamine and Chondroitin are products that apparently are helpful in reducing arthritic pain.

Ginger, generally, is regarded as a safe food supplement by the Food and Drug Administration. It is used in the treatment of nausea and motion sickness and may be taken as a digestive aid. A small study showed the benefit of its use in reducing vomiting during pregnancy. It is safe to try in pregnancy or for motion sickness at 250 mg four times a day.

Ginkgo biloba—There are controversial medical studies regarding its benefit in the improvement of memory, especially in Alzheimer and demented patients. The usual dose is 120–240 mg per day in 2–3 divided doses.

Ginseng can be used in low dosage, such as 900 mg per day, to reduce high blood pressure and improve cases of heart failure. It can increase the effect of Digoxin (a heart medication) and some of the vasodilators (medications that dilate the vessels).

Lycopene is found in tomato sauce. It is considered an antioxidant. It may protect against heart attack or lower the "bad cholesterol" (LDL or low-density lipoprotein). It possibly protects against prostate cancer.

Milk thistle/Silmarin is used in Germany for alcoholic liver disease. It is also worth trying for treatment of amanita mushroom poisoning.

Peanuts are rich in protein, fiber, and several vitamins and minerals. They are packed with a significant amount of resveratol (an antioxidant), which fights against heart attack. There are some indications that peanut butter may reduce the risk of diabetes.

Saw palmetto is a product that has been widely used in patients with enlarged prostate. Apparently, it has weak anti-male hormone activity, which, presumably, reduces the size of the prostate.

St. John's wort is used to treat mild to moderate depression, seasonal affective disorder, and HIV infection. There is not enough data (especially long-term) to recommend its use in combination with other antidepressants due to the potential of added toxicity.

Valerian is suitable for occasional use for insomnia and lowering anxiety. Generally, the FDA considers it as safe.

Herbal products and extracts may interact with prescribed medications. For example, Feverfew, Ginkgo, Garlic and Ginger can increase the risk of bleeding in patients taking aspirin or warfarin (Coumadin®).

V) Love and Relationship

Do you still remember the three layers of the human needs that I described? Love is probably the most important element in the third layer. It is an ultimate emotion for which we all crave. However, is love something you seek out or does it eventually find your heart? Can love grow by itself or will it need your input? Once developed, will love remain in your heart forever or will it fade?

Although contentment does not occur at all times, we were born in order to be happy and remain in that state throughout life. A loving relationship brings happiness. Love is a learned process that is initiated in childhood. A passionate family may teach children how to love and respect others. The establishment of this emotion in an adult relationship is based upon the concepts that people acquired in childhood.

Finding true love in a relationship may not be as hard as you think. The key for opening the door is passion. Love cannot grow or exist on its own. It requires continuous consideration of your partner emotions and an understanding his or her needs. The question remains, what are the priorities and needs that exist in a relationship? In a shared alliance, the basic element is to create an environment that reduces stress and anxiety. This allows for the establishment of emotional stability and the peace of mind of your loved one. An important lesson is to realize that being with someone is a two-way street. It is about giving and taking. The devotion and affection for one another can create trust and a warm relationship, which permits love to grow.

You will have a *good* relationship or marriage when you value your partner's priorities. An *excellent* loving relationship or marriage develops when you set your partner's needs ahead of your own! Obviously, to achieve such a goal is a day-by-day challenge. Be cautious not to make your relationship a disastrous one in which there is no consideration regarding the needs of the other party. In your relationship, into which category do you fall? Can you make it better?

Unfortunately, illnesses and diseases may affect relationships. Many men and women suffer from **impotence** at some time during their lives. For those people, sexual dysfunction and the inability to sexually satisfy their partners may have a great emotional impact. The factors that contribute to sexual dysfunction are multiple. By far, the most important and common factor is of a psychological nature. Stress, anxiety, fatigue, lack of sleep, a low level of affection between partners, and a heavy workload may all affect sexual desire in men and women. Some medications, aging, and certain medical conditions may contribute to erectile dysfunction.

Sildenafil (Viagra®) was introduced to the pharmaceutical market a few years ago. Since then, it has become a successful and effective treatment of men suffering from erectile dysfunction. The upper-most important outgrowth of Viagra®, I believe, was also the creation of a revolution in the way men openly discuss their sexual problems with their physicians. As the media opened the gates of dialogue about this subject, women did not remain behind. They also began expressing to their private practitioners the frustrations of their unsuccessful sexual relationships.

Relaxation, having pleasant conversation with your partner, and taking time off from your busy schedule could be a big step toward coping with and overcoming sexual dysfunction. In some instances, the administration of medications or the use of special devices might be appropriate. Trauma or sexual organ nerve disease, such as in diabetic neuropathy, may cause varying degree of nerve damage. In the severe cases of impairment, medications, such as Viagra®, are probably less helpful.

For some people, the ultimate goal is to be engaged in sexual activity. However, creating a passionate relationship with your partner, including hugging or kissing on a daily basis, can improve your mental and sexual well-being. This can lead to the growth and development of love between the partners. Therefore, starting tomorrow, before you leave your house, don't forget to kiss your partner. Rest assured that the return would be much greater.

The Ten Commands for an Excellent and

a Perfect Marriage

1) Make your spouse the most important person in your life before anybody else.

2) Love and respect your spouse's parents and the family members as is if they are your own.

3) Be honest. Do not lie to each other. This will develop trust between you. Trust will bring love.

4) Do not keep secrets from each other.

5) "Do not bring your dirty clothes to your parent's house". Solve your problems between yourselves. Leave the parents for happy occasions.

6) Have faith in each other's ideas and support each other for a common goal.

7) Have sex with each other—at least twice a week.

8) Never put negative thoughts in each other's head. Always be positive.

9) Never make any threats against or raise your voice on your spouse. Your voice should deliver passion and love.

10) Never raise your hand on your spouse. Your touch should be gentle and a source of comfort.

16

Final Message and Conclusion

Every time I enter a medical library, I see numerous books and journals, indicating the vast scope of the medical field. The various subjects presented in "Passion for Living a Long Life" can serve as "facilitators" for many people to become more educated about taking care of themselves and their dear ones in an ethical and professional manner. Let's learn the take-home messages in the following paragraphs.

Ideology—I wonder if the concept of heaven is true! Humans at large strive hard to have a long life on the Earth. It appears many of us believe there is no life after death. With this notion in mind, I might offend some groups of people who do believe in the "other" world. The controversy, however, remains in place. I assume each individual wants to live on as long as possible, since that person presumes our planet is the ultimate place for living. Therefore, you should seize your one-time chance of existing and develop a healthy pathway to prolong your life.

With new technologies, it seems the heavenly planet Earth, has become smaller. Many cities around the globe assimilate people from different civilizations, thus creating multicultural societies. Destiny brought me to New York, a great metropolis that exemplifies such an atmosphere. One of my patients whose ancestors came to the United States from Holland had a wonderful way of explaining the variations of people. He said, "It is our diversified backgrounds that make our nation strong." I would like to add that it is imperative to respect each different ideology in order to achieve a higher goal—*peace*. This state will develop when every one of us internalizes and accepts the concept of being "different". Peace brings us together. It makes us emotionally stable and promotes new ideas. It is interesting to note that an individual's health is also associated with a peaceful environment in society.

Physicians' responsibilities—Physicians work hard throughout their careers to become valuable sources for helping their patients. During medical school, unlike many other professions, students learn how to utilize their five senses. They must visualize, palpate, listen, smell and, on occasion, even taste, in order to make a diagnosis. Of course, in these modern days, new tools might have reduced the full-scale development of these senses among medical students, but they also increased the physician's aptitude for earlier diagnoses. Yet, nothing can replace the human emotions, which a physician experiences toward a patient.

Visiting a physician may have many meanings for different people. The fear of discovering an abnormality or a disease, or being ashamed of sickness, frequently prohibits some individuals from visiting a doctor for years or even decades. The emphasis for both patients and physicians has to be on preventive medicine. This means learning and implementing ways to avoid diseases.

Good doctors and health professionals listen; the excellent ones interact. The superior ones bring together those skills along with their intelligence and *honesty* to take care of their patients. Many physicians, nurses, physician assistances, nurse practitioners and others in the field of medicine fall into the last category. My recommendation for all of them is to treat your patients as if they were your family members. The key for a successful relation with patients and a superior outcome is a "good intention".

Patients' attitude—As I prepared to unfold the stories in this book, I chose to begin with the tale of a child to indicate the significance of thinking about the next generation—our children. In parallel, we all have a duty toward our bodies and spirit.

Throughout the years, everyone creates recollections which are derived from either enjoyable or unpleasant experiences. These memories are used as skills to improve our existence. Some of these skills enable us to develop our health outlook by shifting detrimental habits to the desired ones. Modifying one's diet to a more appropriate regimen and implementing simple techniques for cardiovascular work out, such as walking distances and using stairs instead of elevators, may go a long way toward extending life. It is hard to renounce old habits, such as smoking, drinking excessive amount of alcohol, or abusing drugs, but the examples in this book may encourage some of you to do so.

For a longer and healthier life, Individuals are advised to follow certain rules. Eating the right food, exercising, and reducing your stress will eventually help you to have a more comfortable life. Using these methods might extend your life span even to one hundred years. I assume, unfortunately, some of us would be demented at this age!

The following table is a summary of some information for longevity. Although this table is controversial in part, it could be a general guideline for healthy living. My suggestion is "do everything in life in moderation".

Appropriate measures for a longer life

Category	Topic	Suggestion
External/ Environ- mental	Annual physical exam	To keep your health in check.
	Medium or large-size car	It protects you from accidents. Do not forget to put your seat belts on while driving. Do not drive under the influence of alcohol, drugs or drowsiness.
Diet and Intake	Proper diet	Low fat, low sugar, and low salt. Reduce the intake of animal proteins.
	Calcium	Total of 1200-1500 mg a day to protect your bones and teeth.
	Red wine	About 3 or 4 glasses a week. Excessive drinking of alcohol causes organ damage, especially to your heart and liver.
	Vitamins	One tablet of multivitamins a day preserves the integrity of your skin, improves your memory, and helps many organs to function properly.
	Don't smoke	Excellent choice! You will save money in the long run as well.
Stress reduction	Sport	At least 20 minutes of exercise 3 times a week. Keeps your heart in shape.
	Sex	At least twice a week! More is welcome!
	Laughter	One of the very important elements -- you need about "3 lbs" of it every day!

◆   ◆   ◆

Throughout my life, I was fortunate to encounter great people who helped me to learn more about the wonders of existence. These were my teachers, colleagues, friends, family members, patients, students and, above all, my parents. All of them were my "facilitators" in my "learning processes" to study, teach, and discover the beauties of life. You may call me Dr. Tabib, or Dr. T, or simply use my nickname Eddie. My message is clear—strive for peace and a healthier, longer life.

APPENDIX A

Medication Index

The following medications have been mentioned in various sections.

Generic name	Brand name
Acarbose	
Alendronate	Fosamax®
Aluminum and Magnesium Hydroxide	Maalox®
Aspirin	
Bromocriptine	
Bupropion	Zyban®
Calcitonin	
Calcium	
Calcium carbonate	Tums®
Carbamazepine	
Chlordiazepoxide	Librium®
Ciprofloxacin	Cipro®
Clonidine	
Clopidogrel	Plavix®
Diazepam	Valium®
Digoxin	
Famotidine	Pepcid AC®
Folic acid	
Haloperidol	

Generic name	Brand name
Heparin	
Hydrochlorothiazide	
Hydrocortisone	
Ibuprofen	Advil®, Motrin®
Lamotrigine	
Metformin	
Miglitol	
Morphine	
Omeprazole	Prilosec®
Oxazepam	Serax®
Penicillin	
Phenobarbital	
Phenytoin	
Raloxifene	Evista®
Ranitidine	Zantac®
Risedronate	Actonel®
Sildenafil	Viagra®
Tamoxifen	Nolvadex®
Teriparatide	Fortèo®
Tetracycline	
Thiamine	
Valproic acid	
Vitamin D	
Vitamin E	
Warfarin	Coumadin®

Herbal Medications

Chondroitin
Echinacea
Feverfew
Garlic (Kwai)
Ginger
Ginkgo biloba
Ginseng
Glucosamine
Lycopene
Milk thistle/Silmarin
Resveratol
Saw palmetto
St. John's wort
Valerian

Appendix B

Directory of Resources

Alcoholic Anonymous—General Service Office   *1-212-870-3400*

Located at 475 Riverside Drive, New York, NY 10115.
Web site: http://www.alcoholics-anonymous.org

Al-Anon/Alateen Family Group Headquarters   *1-800-356-9996*
Canada   *1-800-714-7498*

Located at 1600 Corporate Landing Parkway, Virginia Beech,
VA 23454-5617. It provides free sample of materials.
Web site: http://www.al-anon.alateen.org

American Academy of Addiction Psychiatry   *1-931-341-6680*

Located at 8340 Mission Road, Suite B-4, Prairie Village,
KS 66206.
Web site: http://addicpsych@aol.com

American Academy of Family Physicians   *1-800-274-2237*

Located at 11400 Tomahawk Creek Parkway, KS 66211-
2672.
Web site: http://www.aafp.org

American Academy of Pediatrics   *1-866-THEAAPI*
(1-866-843-2271)
1-847-434-4000

Located at 141 Northwest Point Blvd, Elk Grove Village,
IL 60007-1098.
Web site: http://www.aap.org

American cancer Society, National Hotline   *1-800-ACS-2345*
1-800-227-2345

Local chapters are listed in the white pages of your telephone
book. It provides free information and emotional support
from trained volunteers anytime before, during, or after
treatment. Programs include *Reach to recovery* and *Look
good, Feel better*.

American College of Rheumatology   *1-404-633-3777*

Located at 1800 Century Place, Suite 250, Atlanta,
GA 30345.
Web site: http://www.rheumatology.org

American Diabetic Association   *1-800-DIABETES*
                                                        1-800-342-2383

Located at 1701 North Beauregard Street, Alexandria,
VA 22311.
Web site: http://www.diabetes.org

American Lung Association   *1-800-LUNG-USA*
                                                        (1-800-586-4872)
                                                        1-212-315-8700

Located at 61 Broadway, 6th floor, New York, NY,
10006.
Web site: http://www.lungusa.org

Arthritis Foundation   *1-800-283-7800*

Located at 1330 West Peachtree Street, Atlanta, GA 30309.
The foundation publishes pamphlets, magazines, and
provides up-to-date information on arthritis as research
and treatment, nutrition, and alternative therapies.
Web site: http://www.arthritis.org

Association of Medical Education and Researchers in Substance *1-401-444-1817*
Abuse (AMERSA)

Located at Box G-BH, Brown University, Providence,
RI, 02912.
Web site: http://center.butler.butler.brown.edu/AMERSA/

Betty Ford Center   *1-800-854-9211*
                                                        1-619-773-4100

Located at 39000 Bob Hope Drive, Rancho Mirage,
CA 92270.
Web site http://www.bettyfordcenter.org

Canadian Pediatric Society (CPS)   *1-613-526-9397*

Located at 2204 Walkley Road, Suite 100, Ottawa,
Ontario, K1G 4G8, Canada.
Web site: http://www.cps.ca

CDC Diabetes Public Health Resource   ***1-877-CDC-DIAB***

CDC Division of Diabetes Translation   ***1-877-232-3422***

PO Box 8728, Silver Spring, MD 20910
Web site: http://www.cdc.gov/diabetes

Center for Disease Control and Prevention   ***1-800-311-3435***
1-404-639-3311

Located at 1600 Clifton Road, Atlanta, GA 30333.
Web site: http://www.cdc.gov

Coping: Living with Cancer   ***1-615-791-3859***

A magazine for people living with cancer, whether their
own or that of a friend or family member. Published 6
times annually. P.O. Box 682268, Franklin, TN 37068-2268

Immunization Action Coalition (IAC)   ***1-651-647-9009***

Located at 1573 Selby Ave, Suite 234, St Paul,
MN 55104.
Web site: http://www.immunize.org

Infectious Disease Society of America (IDSA)   ***1-703-299-0200***

Located at 66 Canal Center Plaza, Suite 600, Alexandria,
VA 22314.
Web site: http://www.idsociety.org

Institute of Medicine (IOM)   ***1-202-334-3300***

Located at The National Academies, 500 Fifth St, NW,
Washington, DC 2001.
Web Site: http://www.iom.edu

National Breast Cancer Coalition   ***1-202-296-7477***

Located at 1707 L Street NW, Suite 1060, Washington,
DC 20036. It is a national advocacy group that lobbies
for increased research funding, access to medical
services, and education.
Web site: http://www.natlbcc.org

National Cancer Institute's Cancer Information Hotline   *1-800-4-CANCER*
                                                           (1-800-422-6237)

Offers free state-of-the-art information in English and
Spanish on treatment, clinical trials, eating habits,
advanced cancer, and services in your area.

National Cancer Institute's Office of Alternative Medicine   *1-301-402-2466*

Located at 6120 Executive Blvd., Suite 450, Bethesda,
MD 20892

National Council Against Health Fraud   *1-909-824-4690*

P.O. Box 1276, Loma Linda, CA 92354.
Web site: http://www.hcrc.org

National Diabetes Information Clearinghouse   *1-800-860-8747*

1 Information Way, Bethesda, MD 20892-3560
Web site: http://www.niddk.nih.gov/health/diabetes/ndic.htm

National Fibromyalgia Association   *1-714-921-0150*

Located at 2200 N. Glassell Street, Suite A, Orange,
CA, 92865. This association is concerned with
developing and executing programs dedicated to
improving the quality of life for people with
Fibromyalgia.
Web site: http://www.fmaware.org

National Institute of Health   *1-301-496-4000*

Located at 9000 Rockville Pike, Bethesda, MD 20892.
Web site: http://www.nih.gov

National Osteoporosis Foundation   *1-202-223-2226*

Located at 1232 22nd Street, NW, Washington, DC,
20037-1292
The most updated information about osteoporosis can
be obtained on its web site: http://www.nof.org

National Prostate Cancer Coalition   *1-888-245-9455*
                                        1-202-463-9455

Located at 1154 Street, NW, Washington, DC, 20005
It provides educational materials.
Web site: http://www.pcacoalition.org

National Woman's Health Network   *1-202-347-1140*

Located at 514 10th St, NW, Suite 400, Washington,
DC 20005. It provides newsletters and position papers
on women's health topics

Pediatric Infectious Disease Society   *1-703-299-6764*

Located at 66 Canal Center Plaza, Suite 600, Alexandria,
VA 20001.
Web site: http://www.pids.org

Prostate cancer Research Institute   *1-310-743-2116*

Located at 5777 W. Century Blvd, Suite 885, Los Angeles,
CA 90045. It is a non-profit organization supporting
research and education in prostate cancer

U.S. Food and Drug Administration   *1-888-INFO-FDA*
                                                       1-888-463-6322

Located at 5600 Fishers Lane, Rockville, MD 20857-0001
Web site: http://www.fda.gov

U.S. Food and Drug Administration—Consumer Information Line *1-800-532-4440*

Working hours are 10 AM to 4 PM EST, Monday—Friday.
Record Information

U.S. Food and Drug Administration—HIV/AIDS office of Special *1-301-827-4460*
Health Issues

Web site: http://www.fda.gov/oashi/aids/HIV.html

World Health Organization (WHO)   *(+41 22) 791-21-11*

Located at Avenue Appia 20, 1211 Geneva 27, Switzerland.
Web site: http://www.who.int

Bibliography

The following sources were used in writing the medical materials of this book with granted permission. The author greatly appreciates those publishers for their courteous effort.

(1) New York State Public Health Law—Article 28

(2) Problem Oriented Medical Diagnosis, Harold Friedman, MD, 3rd edition, 1983

(3) Principals of Surgery, Seymor I. Schwart, G. Tom Shires, Frank C. Spencer...[et al], 7th edition, 1999

(4) Textbook of Pulmonary Diseases, Gerald L. Bauman...[et al.], 6th edition, 1998

(5) Essentials of Family Medicine, Philip D. Sloane, et al, 3rd edition, 1998; 527-532

(6) Diabetes Week, August 13, 2001; pNA

(7) FDA Consumer, March-April 2002; 36(2): 7(1)

(8) Harrison's, Principles of Internal Medicine, Eugene Braunwald...[et al.], 15th edition, 2001

(9) National Institute of Health Consensus Conference. Optimal calcium intake: NIH Consensus Development Panel on optimal calcium Intake. JAMA. 1994; 272:1942–1948

(10) Executive Summary of the Third Report of the National Cholesterol Education Program (NCEP) expert panel on detection, evaluation, and treatment of high cholesterol in adults (adult treatment panel III). JAMA. 2001; 285:2486–2497

(11) Current Surgical Diagnosis and Treatment, Lawrence W. Way, 9th edition, 1994, 737–740

(12) Clinical Neurology, Michael Swash and John Oxbury, 1st edition, 1991

(13) General Facts Regarding the Driver—Put the Breaks on Fatalities Day, U.S. Department of Transportation, Federal Highway Administration, October 10, 2001

(14) Red Book, Report of the Committee on Infectious Disease, American Academy of Pediatrics, 25th edition, 2000

(15) Midgley JP, Matthew AG, Greenwood CMT, et al, Effect of reduced dietary sodium on blood pressure. JAMA. 1996; 275:1590–1597

(16) Apple LJ, Moore TJ, Oberzanek E, et al, for the Dietary Approaches to Stop Hypertension Collaborative Research Group. A clinical trial of the effects of dietary patterns on blood pressure. The New England Journal of Medicine 1997; 336:1117–1124

(17) He K, et al, Fish Consumption and Risk of Stroke in Men. JAMA. 2002; 288:3130–3136

(18) The ALLHAT Officers and Coordinators for the ALLHAT Collaborative Research Group, Major Outcomes in High-Risk Hypertensive Patients Randomized to Angiotensin-Converting Enzyme Inhibitor or Calcium Channel Blocker vs Diuretic. The Antihypertensive and Lipid-Lowering Treatment to Prevent Heart Attack Trial (ALLHAT). JAMA. 2002; 288:2981–2997

(19) Glassman AH, Stetner F, Walsh BT, et al, Heavy smokers, smoking cessation and clonidine. JAMA. 1988; 259:2863–2866

(20) Writing Group for the Woman's Health Initiative Investigators, Risk of invasive breast cancer causes early termination of the WHI trial evaluating the long-term use of HRT in postmenopausal women. JAMA. 2002; 288:321–333

(21) Tabibzadeh, F. Basal cell carcinoma of the leg. American Family Physician. 1995; 52(6):1684,1689

(22) Levine B, Smith RA, Feldman GE, et al. Promoting early detection tests for colorectal carcinoma and adenomatous polyps—A framework for action: the strategic plan of the national colorectal cancer roundtable. Cancer. 2002; 95:1618–1628

(23) Harris R. Lohr KN. Screening for prostate cancer: an update of the evidence for the U.S. Preventive Services Task Force. [Review] [164 refs] Annals of Internal Medicine. 2002; 137(11):917–929

(24) Efficacy and Safety of Echinacea in Treating Upper Respiratory Tract Infections in Children. JAMA. 2003; 290:2824–2830

(25) Risk Factors for Advanced Colonic Neoplasia and Hyperplastic Polyps in Asymptomatic Individuals. JAMA. 2003; 290; 2959–2967

About the Author

My medical career began in an ancient country, Iran. I attended the only English language university in that country. As a young, enthusiastic student I had a great opportunity to explore a rich Eastern culture in this setting. While I was deeply involved in social issues, I wrote many articles for a student organization newsletter pertaining to these subjects. However, the path of my education had to be temporarily interrupted when, in 1979, a revolution occurred in Iran. The new public environment, and unfortunately, anti-Semitic waves, did not allow me to continue my medical career in that country. Therefore, I relocated to Israel, where different civilizations and ethnicities mingled with each other. This transition advanced my understanding about human characteristics. On the road toward achieving higher education, I received my Master's degree in microbiology from Tel-Aviv University and, concurrently, I completed the medical school at the Hebrew University in Jerusalem. In order to gain a distinctive experience, I joined the Israeli Defense Army as a physician officer, where I learned how to survive under demanding situations.

I pursued my medical career in the field of family practice in the United States. I became a board certified family physician after graduation from the residency program at the University of Connecticut. By practicing this specialty, I became familiar with a broad spectrum of diseases from pediatric problems to geriatric issues. With such a diverse and rich background, I came to New York, a cosmopolitan city, where I practiced medicine in different settings, such as private office, nursing home, urgent care centers, and hospitals.

By having a deep understanding of issues regarding various ethnicities, I was able to run a multicultural practice of my own in a suburban area of New York City. I followed my patients very closely and became mentally and emotionally involved with them. I recognized the need to educate the community for which I provided medical care. The patients' feedback regarding my care and my past experiences made me believe that there are many others who need to gain more knowledge in medicine in order to have a longer, healthier, and better life.

Over a quarter of a century, either abroad or in the United States, I have encountered many men and women from different nationalities. By treating and caring for them, I have gained much knowledge regarding the unlimited scope of the human character and the varieties of cultures to write *Passion for Living a Long Life*. Throughout these years, I also inherited a nickname, "Eddie Tabib"—a short one for my given name "Farzad Tabibzadeh". It is also utilized as a preferred name in the context of this book.

Address editorial correspondence to:

Farzad Tabibzadeh, MD, MSc
54 Pasture Lane,
Roslyn Heights, NY 11577
E-mail address: ftabib4@msn.com

Index

978-0-595-36044-4
0-595-36044-0